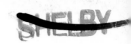

Exercises for
OSTEOPOROSIS

Over 100 Exercises
to Improve Strength, Balance,
and Flexibility

Dianne Daniels, MA

Photography by
Peter Field Peck

HATHERLEIGH PRESS

NEW YORK

A getfitnow.com book

Exercises for Osteoporosis
A Getfitnow.com Book

Hatherleigh Press/Getfitnow.com Books
An Affiliate of W.W. Norton & Company, Inc.
522 46th Avenue Suite 200
Long Island City, NY 11101
1-800-528-2550

Visit our website: www.getfitnow.com

DISCLAIMER: Before beginning any exercise program consult your physician. The authors and publisher of this book and workout disclaim any liability, personal or professional, resulting from the misapplication of any of the training procedures described in this publication.

All Getfitnow.com titles are available for bulk purchase, special promotions, and premiums. For more information, please contact the manager of our Special Sales Department at 1-800-528-2550.

Library of Congress Cataloging-in-Publication Data

Daniels, Dianne.
    Exercises for osteoporosis / Dianne Daniels.
       p.   cm.
    ISBN 1-57826-076-0 (alk. paper)
    1. Osteoporosis—Exercise therapy. I. Title.
    RC931.o73 D53 2000
    616.7'16—dc21   00-037028
                                                            CIP

Cover design by Lisa Fyfe
Text design and composition by John Reinhardt Book Design

Principle photography by Peter Field Peck
with Canon® cameras and lenses on Fuji® slide film

Author photo by Rick McKay

Printed in Canada on acid-free paper
10 9 8 7 6 5 4 3 2 1

DEDICATION

To Bob Deaver, who first planted the seed, and Loretta Lambroussis, who patiently and persistently nourished it.

IN APPRECIATION

To Rebecca Dietzel, who elevated the quality of this book beyond my expectations; to Rick McKay, Julie Simpson, and my parents, who brought the exercises to life; to Amy Eiges and Vicki Beer, who lent their talented voices to the text; and to my wonderful models, Martha Sussman and Paul Frediani, who made it such fun.

Contents

Preface

This book is *not* designed for use without physician guidance. If you have advanced osteoporosis, you are at constant risk of fracture. You may also have other diseases or conditions (e.g. arthritis, heart disease, a hip replacement, etc.) that make specific exercises risky for you. Only your medical team has the knowledge to guide and counsel you with intelligence and safety. This book and the exercises within are *not* intended as a replacement for any course of treatment you are under. Do not stop taking any prescribed medications unless advised to do so by your physician.

CHAPTER ONE

Osteoporosis literally means "porous bone"—a disease
where bone becomes so fragile it is easily broken.

Does Exercise
Really Build Bone?

VERY ONE OF US is at risk for osteoporosis. Regardless of our age,
gender or race, we are all on the osteoporosis continuum. From
the time we are born, our bodies are building bone, the internal
infrastructure that is expected to carry us for the rest of our lives. But
bones reach their peak density in our mid-thirties, and then the inevitable decline begins.

Genetics has the upper hand in the intricate chemistry that deter-
mines the degree and speed with which bone deteriorates. We are
born with certain inherited tendencies that cannot change. Yet with
our future independence and quality of life so drastically threatened
by this disease, is it possible to take a more active role in our own
destiny and ward off these inevitable losses?

We know with certainty that lifestyle plays a crucial role in this
process. For example, we know that smoking, along with what we
eat and drink, dramatically influences bone density. We also know
that people who are active in childhood and continue to exercise in
their adult years have thicker bones. But can we actually "grow" new
bone with exercise begun in adulthood?

1

It has only been in recent years, with advances in modern technology, that we have been able to see, with objectivity and scientific rigor, that exercise *can* make a difference. If you have osteoporosis, exercise may be able to slow down bone loss or put an end to further loss of bone. Simply preventing further decline reduces your risk of fractures and dramatically improves your osteoporosis profile. And in some cases it may be possible for exercise to create *new* bone, perhaps as much as 6%.

If you have been diagnosed with osteoporosis, you probably have lost about 25–35% of desirable bone density. If you've been diagnosed with *osteopenia*, the precursor of osteoporosis, bone loss has been roughly 10–15%. Extensive reviews of the literature conducted by Barbara Drinkwater in 1994[1] and Bernard Gutin in1992[2], two eminent researchers on exercise and osteoporosis, conclude that exercise does *not* increase bone density to the degree necessary to "undo" the losses incurred. In other words, it does not come anywhere near the 25–35% figure.

Fortunately, the effects of exercise are greater than the numbers and statistics would lead us to believe. Exercise can improve your balance, reflexes and coordination, making it less likely you will fall and injure yourself. And with a regular and well-designed exercise routine you can eventually gain the muscle strength and flexibility to catch and protect yourself if you do fall. The importance of these skills can not be stressed enough for someone who, when diagnosed with osteoporosis, lives in constant threat of fracture.

From time to time the media will publicize some new study that claims to build vast amounts of bone. But a single study must be weighed against the total body of research in the field, and some studies are plagued with confounding variables. For example, when some of the subjects in a study perform exercise *and* take an osteoporosis-fighting supplement or drug, the benefits that can be credited to exercise *per se* are scientifically murky. Happily, it appears that exercise *when combined with* your osteoporosis medication has an *additive* effect. So if exercise increases your bone by 2%, and your medication increases it by 5%, then you will have a total net gain of 7% in new bone!

Beginning an exercise program does *not* mean that you can stop taking the medications that have been prescribed to you by your doctor for osteoporosis. But unlike any pill, only exercise can make you stronger, more agile, steadier on your feet, and quicker to react to obstacles in your environment that might cause you to lose your balance and fall. These are perhaps the most compelling reasons to begin an exercise program if you have osteoporosis.

To achieve the reversal of bone loss, exercise must be of a certain type and degree of intensity, and appropriate for your fitness level and fracture risk. Contrary to popular belief, walking does *not* prevent osteoporosis, nor will it build bone, except in the beginning stages of going from couch potato to walker. If you are a non-exerciser and have been relatively sedentary for some time, walking *will* improve bone strength initially, and this is certainly the place to begin your exercise program. However, after a period of time, there is no further benefit from walking alone. The American College of Sports Medicine issued a Position Statement in 1995 putting this myth to rest: "The results from research examining walking . . . demonstrate that this activity, commonly prescribed to postmenopausal women, does *not* prevent bone loss."[3]

Let's examine why. Bone responds to intensity, not duration. In other words, it responds to a force greater than it is used to, not a repetition of the same amount of force. Walking, like all *weight-bearing* activities (running, dancing, skating, etc.), transfers a certain amount of body weight to bones over and over again. At first bone responds by improving its architecture. After a period of time, however, bone acclimates to this level of activity and no longer finds the same amount of exercise a sufficient stimulus for growth.

Enter strength training. This type of exercise, also called *weight training* or *resistance training,* has the ability to progressively and continually challenge bones. It doesn't matter if you use dumbbells, machines, wrist weights, tubing, manual resistance from a partner, or even soup cans—your body has no preference and it doesn't discriminate. When you increase the weight of a dumbbell you use for an exercise, or change to a thicker tubing with greater resistance, you "surprise" the bone and cause it to adapt to this new stress. Bone responds by producing more *osteoblasts,* cells that fill in bone cavities, and bone density improves.

A wonderful study illustrating the need for sufficient resistance in order to improve bone density was conduced on post-menopausal women conducted by Kerr, et al. [4] The researchers had one group of women perform a series of exercises using a weight that allowed them to complete 20 repetitions. Another group did the same exercises, but used a heavier weight so they could only do 8 repetitions. And here's the great touch to the study: both groups only exercised *one* side of their body. The other side, therefore, could act as the *control*, the standard from which to measure the benefit of the exercise. When the results were analyzed only the second group (the one that did the 8 repetition program) increased their bone density, and only on the side that did the exercises.

While this may make you want to go for heavy weight right away, be careful. Begin exercise at a level that is commensurate with your capabilities, and make sure you are able to complete the motion comfortably without any extra weight before adding resistance. Be conscious of your health and medical profile. If you have any injuries, arthritis or joint deterioration, a hip replacement, shoulder, back or knee pain, your exercise program needs to be designed in consultation with your medical team. Heart disease or hypertension might indicate that you need to avoid strenuous weight training. Bear in mind that medications that make you dizzy put you at increased risk of injury (from falling down or dropping a weight) and should influence your exercise choices.

Regardless of any health constraints you may have, just a little exercise can yield significant benefits. In addition to its positive effect on bone, exercise enriches your life by making what you do in the ordinary course of a day so much easier. Carrying groceries, cleaning the home, climbing stairs, picking something up off the floor, or even getting out of a chair don't need to be daunting propositions any more. Improvement may be just around the corner. What you find difficult today can become easy in a matter of weeks.

CHAPTER TWO

The medical costs for osteoporosis are staggering—
$19 million a day, or $7 billion a year.

A Future Epidemic

O STEOPOROSIS IS OFTEN mistakenly perceived of as a disease that only afflicts old women. Most of us will visualize an aged, frail woman, bent over, with a hump on her back. But the reality is quite different. The many faces of osteoporosis include men, as well as women, and young, as well as old.

Disease, alcoholism and steroid use are major causes of osteoporosis in middle-aged and older men. Stringent dieting and over-exercising can result in osteoporosis in young and middle-aged women, a syndrome that even has its own name: the *female athlete triad*. Children and teenagers can lay the groundwork for osteoporosis in later years if they have poor nutrition habits and don't engage in enough physical activity.

It's estimated that osteoporosis affects 25 million Americans, almost 10% of our population. That's one out of every two women, and one out of every five men. And if we don't take preventative steps now, the incidence of osteoporosis is projected to *double* in the next 25 years.

Although these projections can forecast the growing geriatric population, they may actually be *underestimating* future occurrences. For example, both children and adults are spending more and more time sitting in front of computer and television screens, and less and less time in weight-bearing activities. Pre-adolescent girls, easily influenced by society's fears of becoming fat, are beginning to diet as young as seven or eight, reducing their intake of proper nutrients at a critical time in bone development. Additionally, adult women, and men as well, are succumbing to the "thin-is-in" obsession, and developing eating disorders. The dramatic reduction in caloric intake means the loss of vitamins and minerals essential to bone renewal.

The current fad for high protein diets, whether for weight loss or improved athletic performance, also puts bone in jeopardy. These diets cause the body to excrete calcium, a vital component for bone formation. Even the exercise craze has a downside with the desire for bigger and bigger muscles spurring on the use of steroids, a well-known bone antagonist.

There appears to be little doubt that we will see osteoporosis reach epidemic proportions in the near future—if we don't take action. It falls upon each of us, in partnership with our physicians, to seize the initiative and take a vigorous role in our present, and future, health.

CHAPTER THREE

Genetics is thought to account for 70–80% of osteoporosis.
Lifestyle contributes the remaining 20–30%.

Are You at Risk?

THE PART THAT YOU CAN PLAY in your bone's health does have limitations. Regrettably, there is nothing you can do about your age, being a woman, having a small and thin frame, a family history of osteoporosis, or menopause. At the onset of menopause every woman will lose bone because *estrogen*, the female hormone that protects bone, diminishes. But there is much that influences bone that you can control. You may be able to dramatically lower your chances of getting osteoporosis if you avoid smoking cigarettes, drinking large amounts of alcohol, and taking steroids, and if you choose an active lifestyle and balanced diet.

Some prescription and over-the-counter drugs have a harmful effect on bone. Make sure you ask your doctor or pharmacist about the medications that you take. "Boning Up on Osteoporosis," a free publication offered by the National Osteoporosis Foundation, will provide you with a comprehensive overview (*see Appendix B*).

After noting your risk factors for osteoporosis, ask yourself the following evaluative questions:

- **Have I lost any height recently?** A loss of 1″ or more may indicate that you are losing bone.

- **Am I on my feet at least three hours a day?** Spending less time than this does not give bone the minimal stimulus it needs. Extended bed rest due to illness or injury can precipitate osteoporosis.

- **If you are a non-menopausal female: Have I had amenorrhea (loss of menstrual period) for six months or more?** Lack of estrogen is the major cause of osteoporosis in women.

- **If you're an older, thin individual: Does my abdomen extend outward?** This could be an indication that you have already suffered several spinal compression fractures (*see Chapter Four*).

- **Do I have pain in my lower thoracic or lumbar areas (middle back) just to the right or left of my spine?** This is one of the trickiest warning symptoms to be sure of because back pain can be a symptom of many, many other things. And sometimes spinal fractures happen without any back pain at all!

- **Have I had any fractures?** Fractures of the wrist are often the first sign that you have osteoporosis.

- **Have I had any unexplained tooth loss?** Teeth are bones, and losing any could be a sign of severe bone reduction.

- **How's my sex drive?** A decrease in your sex drive can indicate a lower estrogen level in women or testosterone level in men; both are associated with osteoporosis. However, be aware that the nature of your sex drive is complex and a myriad of possible conditions can and do effect it.

If your answers to the above questions suggest you may have osteoporosis, ask your doctor for a *bone densitometry* test. It is painless, harmless, and takes 20 minutes or so. If you're a woman at high risk, it's best to have your first bone density measurement prior to menopause. Don't settle for a regular x-ray—you need to have already lost 20% of your bone for osteoporosis to show up on an x-ray. The preferred test is the one called *dual energy x-ray absorptiometry*, or DXA (also written as DEXA). It will measure the amount of bone you have at one or more of the most common osteoporotic fracture sites and compare you to others of your same gender and age to help you put all the information into perspective.

CHAPTER FOUR

Over a million fractures occur in the United States
each year as a result of osteoporosis.

The Most Common Fracture Sites

A PERSON WITH SEVERE osteoporosis can fracture a bone just by sneezing or being hugged by a loved one. Simple, everyday tasks of lifting a bag of groceries out of the car, opening a window, or bending forward to make a bed can result in a break. About one third of women and nearly one fifth of men will suffer an osteoporosis-related fracture within a normal life span. While these fractures can, and do, occur in any bone of the body, the most common sites are the wrist, spine, and hip.

A wrist fracture is the least debilitating of the three. When it affects the thumb side of the wrist it is called a *Colles'* fracture. In any female over 50, a broken wrist could be an indication that she has osteoporosis.

A decrease in bone density can also affect the bones of the spine, the vertebrae, causing either *compression* or *anterior wedge* fractures. It is possible for several of these fractures to occur in quick succession and cause a woman to lose 4–8 inches of height in only a few months. Surprisingly, these breaks sometimes take place without any appreciable pain.

A protruding stomach on a thin, older woman is another possible indicator of osteoporosis. Repeated spinal fractures may cause two bones—the bottom rib and the top of what is commonly called the hips (anatomically called the pelvic girdle)—to move closer, perhaps even to touch. This lessens the space where internal organs, including the stomach, lie within the torso. With nowhere else to go, the stomach protrudes forward. In addition, people with multiple vertebral fractures are likely to suffer from significantly stooped posture, breathing difficulties, and chronic back pain.

A fall from a standing height is more than twice the force needed to fracture the hip of the average 65 year old. And a hip fracture can be deadly. (While called a hip fracture, the break actually occurs at the top of the thigh bone, the femur). According to the National Osteoporosis Foundation, a woman's risk of getting a hip fracture is equal to the risk of breast, uterine and ovarian cancer combined. And hip fractures due to osteoporosis cause almost as many deaths each year in the United States as do automobile fatalities. Nearly 12–20% of hip fracture victims die from the complications of forced bed rest, such as pneumonia or blood clots that travel to the lungs. And of those survive, about half will lose their ability to live independently.

While this book focuses on the three most common fracture sites, the exercises are far-reaching and will actually benefit most of the bones of the body. It is combination of two forces, the muscles pulling on bones and the direct weight-bearing stresses, that empowers exercise in the fight against osteoporosis.

CHAPTER FIVE

No one knows the exact combination of exercises
that will build bone for *you.*

Why These Exercises
Were Chosen

THIS BOOK FOCUSES on strength, balance and flexibility exercises. Strength exercises have the potential to restore lost bone and to make easier virtually everything you do as you navigate through your daily life. If you've never done strength exercises in the past you will be amazed at how much of a difference they will make.

Good balance enables you to move around with confidence, comfort, and safety. Three bodily systems are at work here. Exercise can improve the *somatosensory* system, which is comprised of tiny neuromuscular receptors in our muscles and joints. Exercise *mobilizes* (or moves) joints and, in so doing, activates these receptors. Occasionally you will see an exercise listed as "mobilization" which means that the joint is being put through a range of motion in order to stimulate its receptors.

Flexibility will add to your ability to readily accomplish daily tasks, to keep your balance, and to be agile. Without adequate flexibility you would find it difficult to get in and out of clothes, to take a bath or a shower, to clean your home, or even to put the groceries away.

As previously mentioned, the focus is on strengthening the bones of the body that are most vulnerable to fractures due to osteoporosis: the spine, the hip, and the wrist.

Exercises for the spine are broken down into those that work the neck, the upper/mid back area, and the lower (or lumbar) area. The entire spine is susceptible because of the type of bone the individual vertebrae are comprised of, namely *trabecular* bone. Therefore, exercises are included to strategically strengthen the entire length of the spine. Of concern to many women with osteoporosis is *kyphosis,* an abnormal outward curve affecting the *thoracic,* or mid-spine, area, which often leads to a bent over body position. If kyphosis is a result of poor posture or muscular weaknesses, it can be greatly improved with targeted strength and flexibility exercises. However, kyphosis that stems from multiple spinal fractures cannot be corrected.

Researchers have looked at the effects of exercise for each of the major osteoporosis fracture sites. It appears to be most difficult to increase bone density for the hip. One exercise that has been shown to be particularly effective is jumping. However, if you would like to include jumping in your program you must do so with great caution, and only with your physician's approval.

In addition to strength, balance, and flexibility exercises, you'll see several other sections:

- **Torso stabilization exercises** simultaneously strengthen all the muscles of the torso, including the abdominals and the *erector spinae* (the collective name for the many muscles attaching along your spine). This can give you the ability to prevent yourself from falling if someone accidentally bumps into you.

- **Exercises for the chest and the arms** will add to your ability to function in your daily life because so many things you do, such as carrying groceries or cleaning your home, require upper body strength.

- **Abdominal exercises** are included because these muscles help keep you in an upright posture. The deepest layer of the four abdominal muscles are the *transverse abdominus.* They support the internal organs lying within the abdominal cavity. The *rectus abdominus,* especially when strengthened in their *eccentric,* or lowering, function, help us to regain posture should we become off-balance. *Kegels,* the movement that engages the muscles of the pelvic floor, are incorporated into the abdominal section.

These will also help to support the internal organs and may play a role in preventing urinary incontinence.

■ **Balance** exercises use the whole body, but particularly the lower leg. Shifting your weight from side to side, standing on one foot, and moving your upper and lower body in opposition are some tactics to improve balance. Research shows that people with weak *anterior tibialis* muscles (the muscles which run along your shins), tend to fall more often. A history of falls is also associated with weak inner thigh muscles (*hip adductors*), front thigh muscles (*quadriceps*), and back thigh muscles (*hamstrings*), all of which are targeted in the "Hip" exercise series. So when you strengthen and stretch *any* of your leg muscles you are helping to maintain or improve balance.

■ **Breathing** is vital for life. Therefore, it makes sense to strengthen the muscles used in breathing. Deep breathing expands the normal movement of the ribcage (which has a tendency to become rigid with age), "massages" the internal organs, and even increases your energy by allowing you to take in more oxygen.

Aerobic activities are certainly very important; they are "heart healthy", help to maintain a good body weight, improve mood, increase longevity, and have many other positive outcomes. Weight-bearing aerobic exercise is the most beneficial type of aerobic activity for osteoporosis because your body weight is being supported by your bony structure. The glaring example of an aerobic activity that does *not* fall into this category is swimming. While swimming is a great aerobic exercise, and you should feel free to incorporate it into your exercise program, if you are striving to build bone, don't make it your *only* aerobic activity.

Weight-bearing aerobic exercise should be part of your strategy for fighting osteoporosis. Walking is easy to do almost anywhere and costs nothing. You can enhance its bone-building value by wearing a backpack into which you progressively, over time, insert weights. These additional loads are transmitted to your spine and hips and, perhaps, can cause bone improvement. If you have severe spinal osteoporosis or kyphosis, you may want to consider, after medical consultation of course, using a weighted belt around your waist, rather than a backpack. (*see Appendix A*)

CHAPTER SIX

An exercise that is safe for one person
may not be safe for another.

Exercise Precautions

THERE IS NO WAY for a book to tell what is beneficial, or what is harmful, for you. Therefore, *you must get clearance from your physician before undertaking any of these suggestions or specific exercises.* Show your doctor the exercises you would like to do and ask if they are suitable given your specific set of circumstances. If you had had a hip replacement or previous surgery, or if you suffer from chronic pain in any of your joints, some exercises may not be right for you. If you have any chronic disease or condition, you may be advised to limit your range of activities.

When exercising, remind yourself of the following:

■ **Exercise should be pain-free**. There is a simple axiom to follow: "If it hurts, don't do it." Often this will mean you need to work in a partial range of motion. There is normal discomfort from working muscles when you begin an exercise program. *Delayed onset muscle soreness* can emerge one or two days after your exercise session. You must become an interpreter of your body's signals to learn what is normal, and what is not, to distinguish between something that is hard to do and something that hurts. Generally, you should not experience any pain in

15

your joints. Joint pain that persists needs to be medically evaluated. Pain in a muscle, however, can be the normal result of stress from exercise. However, if the pain lasts more than a couple of days it may signal other conditions, such as muscle strain, and merits a doctor's visit. Failure to comfortably put weight on a limb, numbness, tingling, or a "pins and needles" sensation require immediate attention.

- **Keep breathing**. Most of us have a tendency to hold our breath when performing challenging exercises. For anyone with hypertension or heart disease, this is medically unwise. Pay special attention when performing exercises where you are required to hold a position for a few seconds.

- **Watch out for shoulder and neck tension**. Take a deep breath, and as you exhale, feel the shoulders relax and the stiffness in your neck melt away.

- **Maintain good neck alignment**. When lying on your back you may need to place small pillow under your head to avoid arching your neck.

- **Hold weights with a neutral wrist**. Place your palms and forearms on a flat surface and note the alignment of your wrist. When you hold any type of weight or tubing do not let your wrist bend backwards, which many people will tend to do. Over time, this puts your wrist joint, and the muscles and tendons running through it, at risk for conditions such as carpal tunnel syndrome.

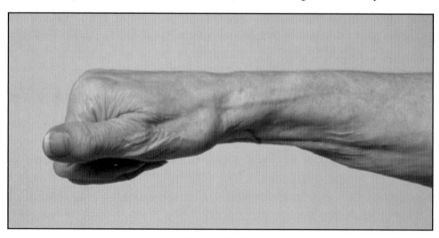

Neutral Wrist

■ **Maintain your normal spinal curves.** A common misconception is that if you "flatten your spine," "tuck your pelvis under," or "press your back down" you protect your back from injury. Nothing could be further from the truth. Changing the configuration of your spine makes it *less* protective, and more prone to initiating back problems. The key is to engage your abdominals during every exercise.

■ **Evaluate your hand grip.** If objects have a tendency to fall from your grasp, strap on wrist weights instead of holding a dumbbell or other exercise equipment. Anyone with severe osteoporosis may want to *always* use wrist weights as a safer alternative.

■ **Avoid forward bending.** None of the exercises in this book cause your trunk to bend forward, which increases your risk of spinal fracture. Evaluate any other exercises or daily activities you perform to avoid this potentially harmful movement.

CHAPTER SEVEN

There may be a fine line between exercise that causes a fracture, and exercise that increases bone density.

The Exercise Program

THERE ARE SIX SAMPLE exercise programs that you can follow, or you can choose exercises *a la carte*. If doing the latter, be sure to select at least one exercise from each category. You may focus on specific areas, but structure your sessions so they are balanced and work your entire body. In general, the exercises in each chapter proceed from easiest to most difficult. Flexibility exercises are included at the end of each strength chapter.

The osteoporosis programs are designed for individuals who have minimal strength, flexibility and balance. Program 1 can be done sitting or lying in bed and requires no special equipment. Program 2 includes the use of a dynaband. As you progress, dumbbells and ankle weights can be added to increase the intensity of the exercises.

Before undertaking either the Osteopenia or Prevention programs, be sure you can easily accomplish the exercises listed in the Osteoporosis programs. If you have a partner, or a personal trainer, try the second program in each category.

In you need to purchase the equipment used in this book, see *Appendix A*. Soup cans, or other household items, can be used instead of dumbbells. Check the label to see how much they weigh. You may begin with 6–8 ounces (about ½ pound). For a stick to use in the exercises called "Battle" you can use part of a broom. If you do not wish to purchase the stepping bench illustrated in the pictures, use the bottom step of a flight of stairs in your home or apartment building.

You will achieve maximum safety and effectiveness by following these simple guidelines.

- **Do a general warm-up**. Prior to doing any of the specific strength or flexibility exercise, do an activity for 5–15 minutes that will gradually elevate your body temperature and heart rate. This gets your muscles primed and ready to undertake the challenge of resistance training. Depending on your fitness level, any type of aerobics can fit the bill. For example, you can warm up on a bicycle, treadmill, Stairmaster, Nordic Track, or rowing machine. If you do not have access to this type of equipment just march in place, gradually lifting your knees higher while increasing the swing of your arms.

- **Do a specific warm-up**. Perform any strength exercise you are planning to do *without* resistance first. Do the movement at least 10 times. This gets a substance called *synovial fluid* to flow and lubricate the joints before you add the intensity of weights.

- **Beginners start with no weights or light weights**. If an exercise is challenging without holding a dumbbell or strapping on an ankle weight, then this is the place for you to start. Progress to using a weight that allows you to do 15 repetitions of the exercise. Rest for 30–60 seconds, and then repeat. In this case it means you will be doing *2 sets of 15 reps*. All beginners should start with lighter weights and more repetitions.

- **Your goal is heavy weights**. Remember that bone responds to how hard you work, not how much. It's better from bone's perspective to use a weight that allows you to do only 6-8 repetitions than to perform 15 repetitions with a lighter weight. Your osteoporosis-fighting strategy is to chose a weight that allows you to do only 6–8 reps of an exercise (after which it is too heavy for you to move). *Do 2 sets of 6–8 reps*. Take a *60 second* rest period between sets.

- **Progress over time**. Over time you need to gradually increase the amount of resistance. When you can do 15 repetitions of a specific exercise with a given resistance, increase the weight. With dumbbells, use increments of ½ pound if you are a beginner or if you have osteoporosis. If you have osteogenia or are disease-free, you may, if approved by your doctor, increase by one pound. When you can do 15 repetitions of a specific exercise, increase the weight. Build up using this new weight over a period of time, until you can do 15 repetitions. Then increase the amount of weight again. It can take days, weeks, or months to increase by even one pound. Take your time, go slow, and do what is right for *you*.

- **Do exercises slowly**. Performing exercises quickly uses momentum, not muscles. Your speed should allow you to easily pause the movement at any point. An added benefit of taking your time is that you are less likely to cause an injury.

- **Rest one to two days between strength workouts**. After an exercise session that includes a strength component, muscles need 24–48 hours to recover. Therefore, always have at least one day of rest before you undertake this type of workout again. Ideally, you should devote 2–3 sessions per week to strength training.

- **Flexibility exercises can be done every day**. Ease into each stretch until you feel a gentle pull. Hold the stretch at this point for a slow count of 15. Take a breath and then as you exhale increase the stretch just a little bit. Hold the stretch again for a slow count of 15.

- **Work both sides**. Although it is not generally indicated in the exercise descriptions, remember that all exercises should be done on the right *and* the left sides of your body.

- **Complete all repetitions on one side first**. Unless indicated otherwise, keep repeating the exercise on one side before switching to the other side.

- **Note your muscular imbalances**. As you do the exercises pay attention to any differences in strength and flexibility between the two sides of your body. These differences are specific to each exercise and to each muscle. Is one arm or leg noticeably weaker when you do a specific exercise? Then do one extra set of the exercise just for that side. Is one arm or leg less flexible than the other? Then give it an extra stretch.

- **Vary your program**. From time to time, change the exercises you do. Remember that bone responds to surprise.

21

CHAPTER EIGHT

Exercises

Resisted Neck #1

· STRENGTH ·

SPLENIUS CAPITIS, SPLENIUS CERVICIS, ERECTOR SPINAE,
SEMISPINALIS CERVICIS, SEMISPINALIS CAPITIS

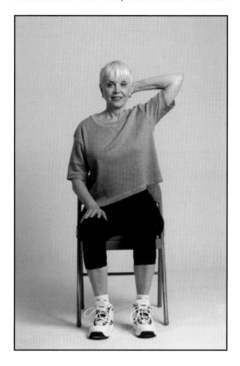

Place a hand on back of your skull. Use the muscles on the back of the neck to press the neck into the hand. Resist with the hand so that no movement actually occurs although you feel the muscles in the back of the neck working. Hold for a count of 3, then release.

- The neck is a particularly vulnerable area. Do not do any neck exercise that causes you pain.
- Lightly stroke the muscles along the back and side of the neck to "wake up" the muscles which will perform the exercise.
- Move the head against the hand first. Resist with the hand second. If done in reverse order you may irritate any arthritis in the neck.
- Continue to challenge yourself by using more hand pressure.
- Keep breathing normally throughout the exercise.

Resisted Neck #2

· STRENGTH ·

STERNOCLEIDOMASTOID, LONGUS COLLI, LONGUS CAPITIS,
RECTUS CAPITIS ANTERIOR, RECTUS CAPITIS LATERALIS

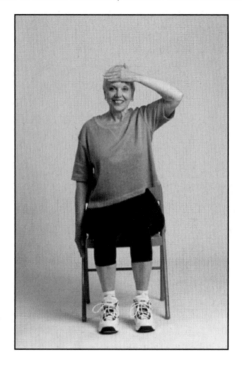

Place a hand on your forehead. Use the muscles on the front of the neck to press the neck into the hand. Resist with the hand so that no movement actually occurs although you feel tension developing in the front of the neck. Hold for a count of 3, then release.

- Lightly stroke the muscles along the front of the neck to "wake up" the muscles which will perform the exercise.
- Move the head against the hand first. Resist with the hand second.
- Increase the difficulty by pressing more with your hand.
- Remember to keep breathing.

26

Resisted Neck #3

· **STRENGTH** ·

STERNOCLEIDOMASTOID, SCALENI, SPLENIUS CAPITIS, SPLENIUS CERVICIS, ERECTOR
SPINAE, SEMISPINALIS CERVICIS, SEMISPINALIS CAPITIS

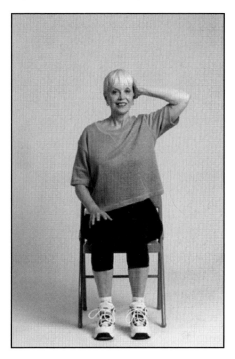

Place a hand on left side of your head. Use the muscles on the left side of
the neck to press the neck into the hand. Resist with the hand so that no
movement actually occurs although you feel tension developing in the
neck muscles. Hold for a count of 3, then release. Do all repetitions and
then switch to the right side.

- Lightly stroke the muscles along the side of the neck to "wake
  up" the muscles which will perform the exercise.
- Activate the muscles first. Resist with the hand second.
- Continue to challenge yourself by using more hand pressure.

Head Lift Side

· STRENGTH ·

STERNOCLEIDOMASTOID, SCALENI, SPLENIUS CAPITIS, SPLENIUS CERVICIS, ERECTOR
SPINAE, SEMISPINALIS CERVICIS, SEMISPINALIS CAPITIS

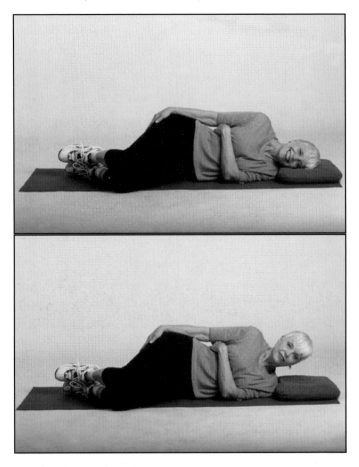

Lie on your right side in a relaxed position with your head on a towel or small pillow. Lift head up as if to place left ear on the left shoulder and then lower slowly. Complete all repetitions and then perform on your left side.

- Avoid movement of the shoulders and torso. Lift the head only.
- Do not push or pull with your arms.

Head Lift Back

• STRENGTH •

SPLENIUS CAPITIS, SPLENIUS CERVICIS, ERECTOR SPINAE,
SEMISPINALIS CERVICIS, SEMISPINALIS CAPITIS

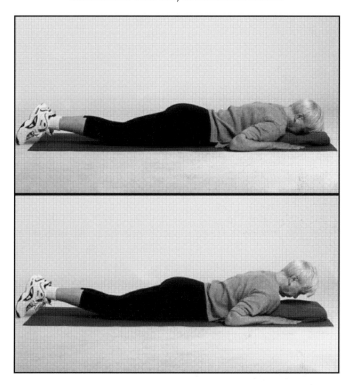

Lie on your stomach and place your chin on a pillow, if comfortable.
Think of reaching out through the top of your head with a long neck as
you lift head off the floor. Pause, slowly lower.

- Do not perform this exercise if you are uncomfortable lying on
  your stomach.
- Keep your shoulders and chest on the floor.
- Avoid pushing with your arms.

Head Lift Front

· **STRENGTH** ·

RECTUS ABDOMINUS, INTERNAL AND EXTERNAL OBLIQUES, STERNOCLEIDOMASTOID, LONGUS COLLI, LONGUS CAPITIS, RECTUS CAPITIS ANTERIOR, RECTUS CAPITIS LATERALIS

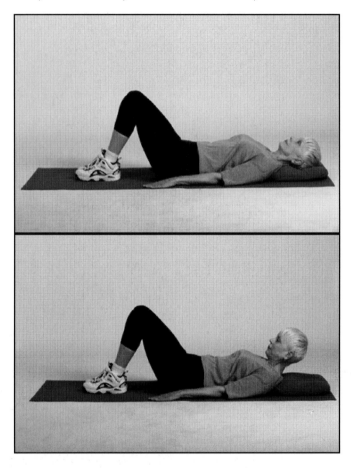

Lie on your back. Tighten your abdominals and think of bringing your chin to your chest as you lift up your head. Pause, lower slowly.

- Do not perform this exercise if you have severe kyphosis.
- Your upper back remains on the floor. Move only your head.
- Begin with just bringing your chin to your chest without lifting up your head at all.
- Progress to leading with your chin as you lift your head up.

Neck Rotation

· FLEXIBILITY / MOBILIZATION ·

LONGUS COLLI, LONGUS CAPITIS, RECTUS CAPITIS ANTERIOR, RECTUS CAPITIS LATERALIS, SPLENIUS CAPITIS, SPLENIUS CERVICIS, ERECTOR SPINAE

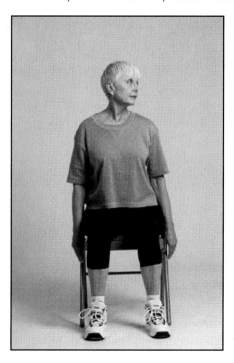

Look straight ahead. Lead with your eyes as you turn your head to look over your right shoulder as far as you can with comfort. Return to starting position. Repeat all repetitions to the right and then perform to the left side.

■ As you look to the right, keep your left shoulder down. You can gently touch the left shoulder as a cue to relax.

■ Do not rotate the torso. Movement is in the neck only.

Retraction

· STRENGTH ·

RHOMBOIDS, MIDDLE TRAPEZIUS

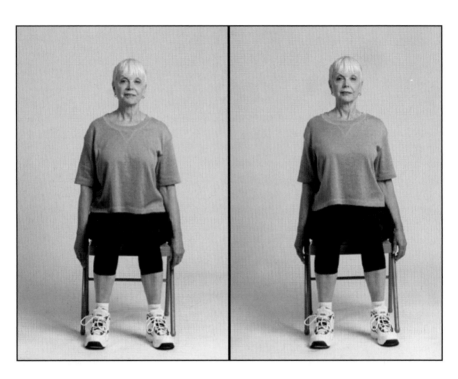

Bring your shoulder blades together. Keep your arms relaxed so that you initiate movement with the muscles between the shoulder blades.

- Maintain a straight and long spine.
- When you can do 2 sets of 12 reps each, progress to "Bent Arm Retraction."

Bent Arm Retraction

• STRENGTH •

RHOMBOIDS, MIDDLE TRAPEZIUS, DELTOIDS, SUPRASPINATUS, SUBSCAPULARIS

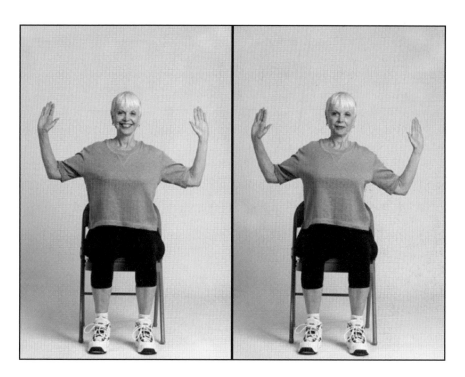

Hold your arms so that they form a 90° angle (goal post arms). Now bring your shoulder blades together, pause, release gently.

■ Keep your spine erect and elongated.
■ Initiate the movement with the muscles between the shoulder blades, not with the arms.
■ Do not let shoulders come up toward the ears.
■ Keep the arms up so the elbows do not drop with the movement.
■ When you can do 2 sets of 12 reps each, progress to "Row with Dynaband."

Row with Dynaband

• STRENGTH •

LATISSIMUS DORSI, POSTERIOR DELTOIDS, BICEPS

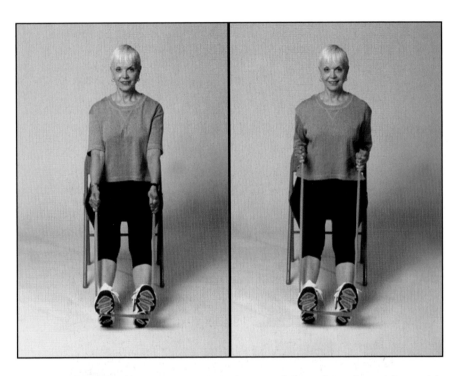

Sit on a chair and secure a dynaband around the soles of your feet with your legs comfortably extended. Hold one end of the band in each hand, thumbs facing up. Keep an erect posture, chest up and abdominals engaged as you pull the band back as far as you can, letting the elbows go behind your torso. Pause, then release slowly.

- Don't let the dynaband "snap back" or "go slack" at any time.
- Adjust the length of the tubing, or switch to a thicker one, so that you get an appropriate challenge.
- Avoid any forward, backward, or twisting movement of the torso. Keep your chest up so that your spine stays lengthened and straight.
- Shoulders stay relaxed and facing forward.

Reverse Fly with Dynaband

· STRENGTH ·

LATISSIMUS DORSI, MID-TRAPEZIUS, RHOMBOIDS, POSTERIOR DELTOIDS

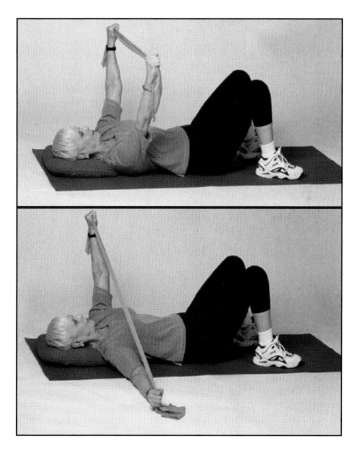

Lie on your back. Place the soles of your feet on the floor. Hold a dynaband or tubing out in front of your body over the mid chest area. Keep your elbows straight as you pull one end of tubing toward your side as far as possible. Pause, release slowly.

■ Keep the movement over your mid chest and not over your neck.
■ The elbow does not bend at all as you pull.
■ Control the tension in the band so it does not go slack or snap back.
■ Maintain a neutral wrist position. Avoid the tendency of the wrist to bend backwards as you pull.

Side Reverse Fly

· STRENGTH / STABILIZATION ·

LATISSIMUS DORSI, MID-TRAPEZIUS, RHOMBOIDS, POSTERIOR DELTOIDS

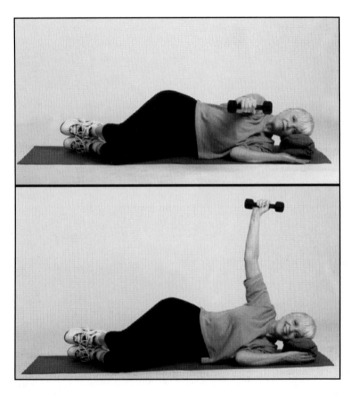

Lie on your right side in a comfortable position with your knees bent. Your left arm will be straight out in front of you so that your hand is about 6 inches off the floor. Lift your arm toward the ceiling until it is perpedicular to your body (and no further). Feel the shoulder blade move toward the middle of your back. Lower slowly to starting position.

- Do not allow your body to rock back and forth. Stabilize by using your abdominals.
- Keep your arm level to the shoulder joint. Avoid letting it move towards your torso, which it will have a tendency to do.
- Maintain a lengthened spine with your chest lifted.

36

Superman

· STRENGTH ·

UPPER, MIDDLE, AND LOWER TRAPEZIUS, POSTERIOR DELTOIDS, SERRATUS ANTERIOR

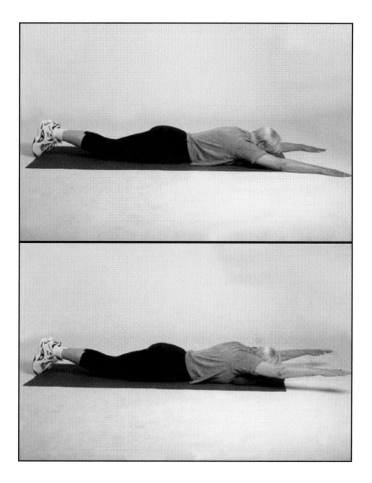

Lie face down. Place your head in a comfortable position (try placing your forehead on the floor). Reach both arms overhead (like superman flying). Lift both arms off the floor, pause, then lower slowly.

- If you have curvature of the spine, as with advanced spinal osteoporosis, place a pillow under your chest.
- Avoid bending your elbows as you lift your arms.
- Begin with no weight. When you can perform 15 repetitions, add a ½ pound dumbbell in each hand.

Goal Post

• STRENGTH •

LATISSIMUS DORSI, RHOMBOIDS, MID-TRAPEZIUS, POSTERIOR DELTOIDS, INFRASPINATUS, TERES MINOR

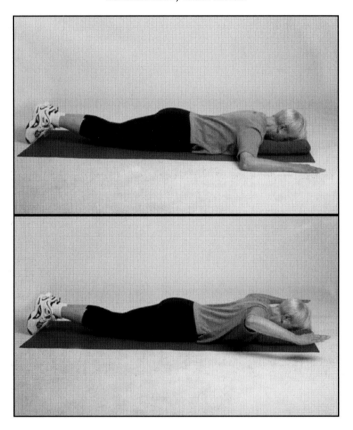

Lie face down. If comfortable, place your forehead on the floor. If not, turn your head to one side, or try a pillow under your chest. Bend your arms at 90° angles (to resemble goal posts). Lift the arms off the floor as high as you can. Pause, lower slowly.

- If you have curvature of the spine, as with advanced spinal osteoporosis, place a pillow under your chest.
- Do not allow the elbows to drop down below shoulder level.
- When you can perform 15 repetitions, progress to holding a ½ pound dumbbell in each hand.

Spine Press

· **STRENGTH** ·

ERECTOR SPINAE

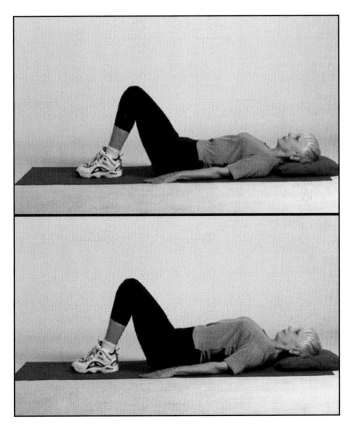

Lie on your back with your head resting on a pillow. Press your head into the pillow and feel your chest begin to lift up off the floor.

- Your head does move. Simply press right where the back of your head rests on the pillow.
- Avoid the tendency to hold the breath. Exhale as you press, and inhale as you return to starting position.

Modified Trunk Lift

· STRENGTH ·

ERECTOR SPINAE

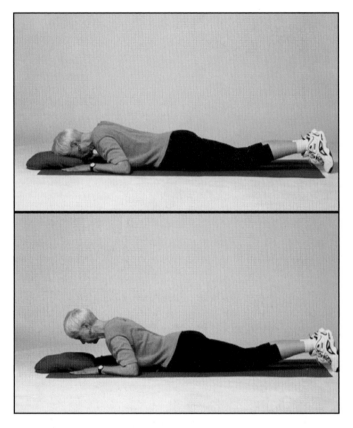

On your stomach, head resting comfortably. Place your forearms on the floor, elbows close to your sides, palms down. Engage your abdominals and press the hip bones into the floor. Bring your head, upper back, and then mid back off the floor, until you feel the contraction of the muscles in the lower back. You can press down with your arms to assist with the extension. Pause, then lower slowly in reverse order.

- You may place a pillow under your abdominal area for comfort.
- Try to minimize the involvement of the muscles in your buttocks and legs. Focus on feeling the muscles in the lumbar spine (lower back) doing the work.
- Be sure to keep breathing.

Hip Walks

• STRENGTH •

QUADRATUS LUMBORUM, OBLIQUES, ERECTOR SPINAE

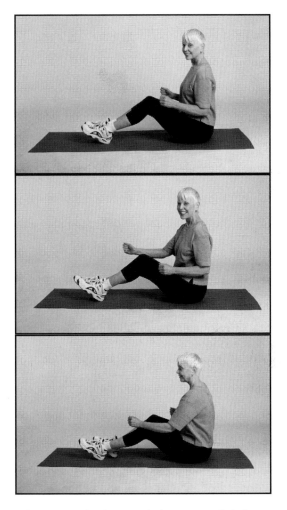

Sit on a mat. Lift your right hip and then your left hip up so that you "walk" forward. Aim for 10 "walks" forward and 10 "walks" backward.

41

Arm and Leg Raise

· STRENGTH ·

ERECTOR SPINAE, GLUTEUS MAXIMUS, HAMSTRINGS, DELTOIDS, TRAPEZIUS

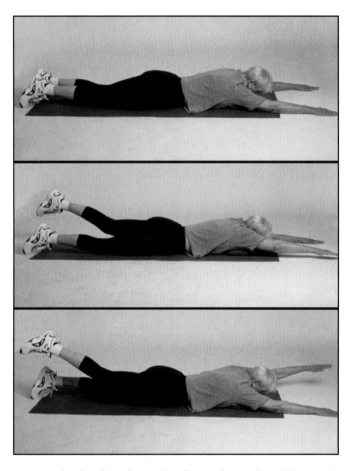

On your stomach, forehead on the floor if comfortable, and arms extended overhead. While pressing both hip bones into the floor, lift up your right leg and left arm. Hold for 5 seconds. Change sides.

- Keep your buttocks and legs muscles relaxed. Focus on feeling the lower back working.
- Progress to performing this exercise with wrist and ankle weights.
- A further progression is using a stability ball (see next exercise).

Arm and Leg Raise with Stability Ball

· STRENGTH / STABILIZATION ·

ERECTOR SPINAE, GLUTEUS MAXIMUS, HAMSTRINGS, DELTOIDS, TRAPEZIUS

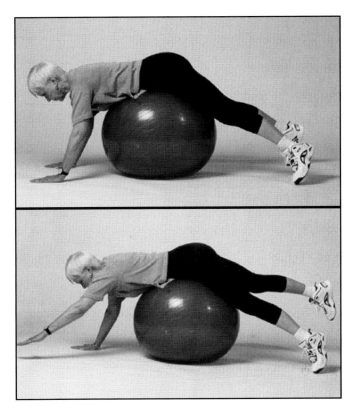

Place your torso over the stability ball as you straighten your legs. Lift up your right arm and left leg. Hold for 5 seconds. Change sides.

■ Adjust how you are positioned over the ball so that you are challenged appropriately.

■ You may begin by just lifting one leg at a time (without the arm), and by just lifting one arm at a time (without the leg).

■ Focus on feeling the muscles in your lower back working while reaching your legs and arms out long.

■ Progress to using wrist and ankle weights.

Four Point Arm and Leg Raise

· STRENGTH ·

ERECTOR SPINAE, GLUTEUS MAXIMUS, HAMSTRINGS, DELTOIDS,
TRAPEZIUS, ABDOMINALS

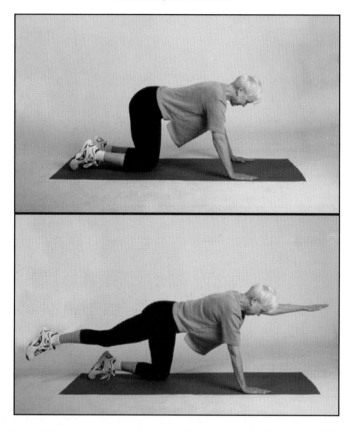

On hands and knees, extend your right leg out in back and lift it up a few inches off the floor. Then straighten your left arm up in front of you and lift it up a few inches off the floor. Your goal is to hold this position for 10 seconds, without wobbling or letting the arm or leg move.

- Focus on feeling the lower back working to keep you stable.
- Maintain a neutral spine, i.e. no sagging in the middle, by keeping your abdominals lifted up.
- Over time aim to get both the arm and the leg parallel to the floor.
- Progress to performing this exercise with wrist and ankle weights.

44

Trunk Lift with Stability Ball

· STRENGTH ·

ERECTOR SPINAE

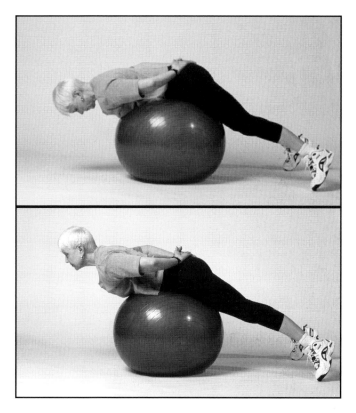

Place your stomach over a stability ball (if uncomfortable, rest your hands on the ball). Lift your body in an arc, beginning with your head, then upper back, then lower back. Pause, then lower in reverse order.

- Initially do this exercise with the soles of your feet pressed against a wall.
- Focus on using the muscles in your lumbar spine to do this exercise rather than the muscles in your buttocks and legs.
- Adjust the position of the stability ball to give you adequate challenge.
- Increase intensity by using "superman arms."

Walking with Rotation

• FLEXIBILITY / BALANCE / COORDINATION •

THE WHOLE BODY

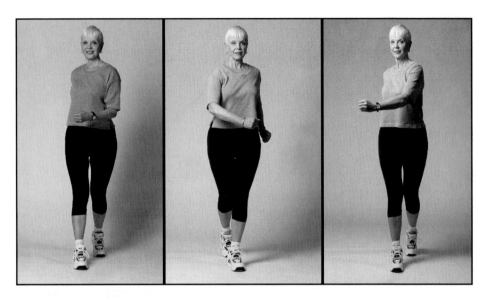

Hold your arms up with bent elbows near your sides. Take a step forward with your right foot and twist your torso to the right. Then take a step forward with your left foot and twist your torso to the left. Let your body move in the direction you are turning to, and relax your lower trunk and pelvis.

Knee to Chest

• FLEXIBILITY •

ERECTOR SPINAE, GLUTEUS MAXIMUS, HAMSTRINGS

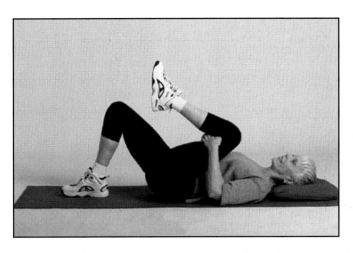

Lie on your back, soles of both feet flat on the floor. Bring your left knee into your chest. Place both hands around the back of the left leg. Inhale, and as you exhale pull the leg in closer to your chest. Hold for 15 seconds. Slowly return to starting position. Perform with other leg.

Bridge

· STRENGTH / STABILIZATION ·

GLUTEUS MAXIMUS, HAMSTRINGS, QUADRICEPS, ERECTOR SPINAE, ABDOMINALS

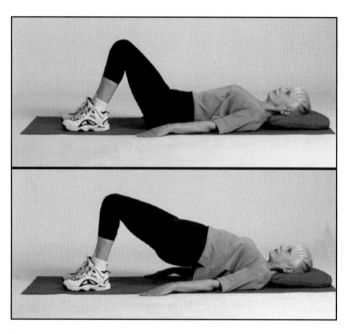

Lie on your back with your knees bent and the soles of your feet on the floor. Activate your abdominals by pulling your navel in towards your spine without pressing your lower back down. Now maintain this position of the spine as you lift your hips off the floor as high as possible. Pause, then slowly lower.

- You may aggravate your sacroilliac joints and cause lower back pain if you fail to maintain abdominal control.
- Do not tuck your pelvis under as you raise up.
- Your hip bones should remain level (one should not be lower than the other) throughout the exercise.
- To increase intensity, add one weight near each of your hip bones (anywhere that's comfortable).
- When you can perform this exercise with your hips bones perfectly aligned while raising and lowering, you may progress to "One-Legged Bridge."

One-Legged Bridge

• STRENGTH / STABILIZATION •

GLUTEUS MAXIMUS, HAMSTRINGS, QUADRICEPS, ERECTOR SPINAE,
RECTUS ABDOMINUS, OBLIQUES

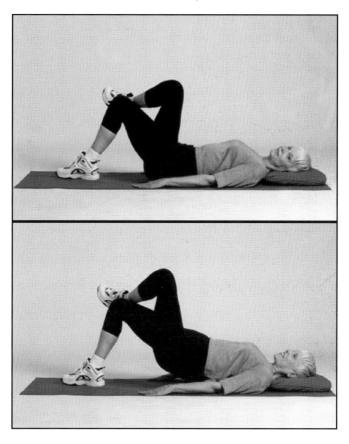

Lie on your back with your left foot on the floor and right leg crossed over the left thigh. Contract your abdominals but do not flatten your spine or tuck your pelvis under. Now lift your hips off the floor as high as possible, keeping both hip bones level. Lower slowly, still keeping your right and left hips in line.

- Do not let the hip of the crossed over leg dip below the level of the other hip.
- To increase intensity, add weight over the hip of the leg on the floor.

Bridge with Stability Ball

· STRENGTH / STABILIZATION ·

GLUTEUS MAXIMUS, HAMSTRINGS, QUADRICEPS, ERECTOR SPINAE, ABDOMINALS

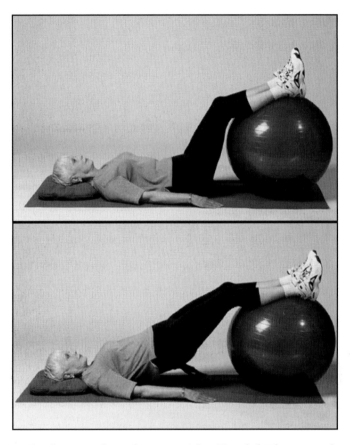

Lie on your back, arms down by your sides. Bend the knees and rest your legs comfortably over a stability ball. Activate your abdominals by strongly pulling your navel in towards your spine. Lift your hips off the floor as high as possible, then slowly lower.

- Your goal is to perform the entire movement with your right and left hip bones evenly aligned (one hip bone should not dip lower than the other).
- For added challenge, cross your arms over your chest.

Pelvic Stabilization

· STRENGTH / STABILIZATION ·

RECTUS ABDOMINUS, INTERNAL AND EXTERNAL OBLIQUES,
ERECTOR SPINAE, HIP FLEXORS

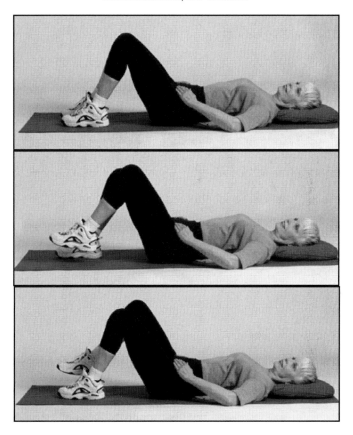

Lie on your back with the soles of your feet on the floor. Place your hands over your hip bones. Pull your abdominals in strongly. Without letting the hip bones move to either side, lift the right foot one inch off the floor, then place the right foot down and lift up your left foot.

- Pretend you have a stick over your hip bones. The stick should not tilt as you switch feet.
- Only lift the foot up 1-2 inches (the foot barely comes off the floor).
- You should really feel the abdominals working if you are doing this exercise correctly.

Pelvic Stabilization with Bridge

• STRENGTH / STABILIZATION •

RECTUS ABDOMINUS, INTERNAL AND EXTERNAL OBLIQUES, ERECTOR SPINAE,
GLUTEUS MAXIMUS, HIP FLEXORS, QUADRICEPS

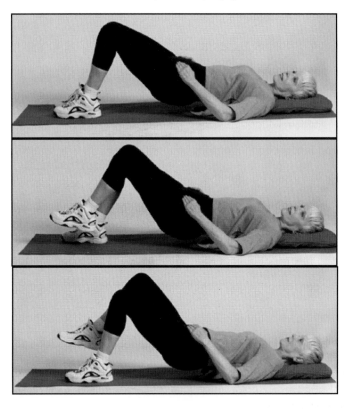

Lie on your back with the soles of your feet on the floor. Place your hands over your hip bones. Pull your abdominals in. Bring your buttocks off the floor as high as you can with comfort. Without letting the hip bones move to either side, lift your right foot one inch off the floor, lower it, then lift up your left foot, then lower it. Your challenge is not to let the hip bones move at all as you switch feet.

■ Do not attempt this exercise until you can easily perform "Pelvic Stabilization."

■ The buttocks do not move at all. They remain lifted up and do not tilt to either side.

■ You are only lifting the foot up one inch so the foot barely comes off the floor.

Partner Push #1

· STRENGTH / STABILIZATION ·

ERECTOR SPINAE

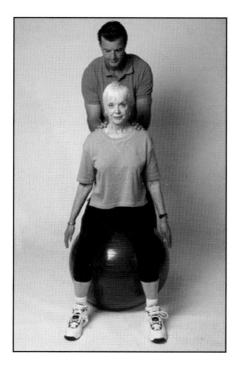

Sit on a stability ball with your arms hanging down by your sides. A partner places his or her hands on your upper back. Resist as your partner gently tries to push you forward.

- Avoid using your arms, hands or legs. Focus on the muscles of your torso.
- Have your partner increase and decrease pressure slowly.

53

Partner Push #2

· STRENGTH / STABILIZATION ·

RECTUS ABDOMINUS, INTERNAL AND EXTERNAL OBLIQUES, TRANSVERSE ABDOMINUS

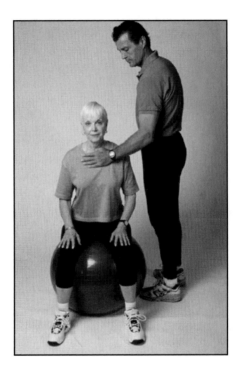

Sit on a stability ball with your arms hanging down by your sides. A partner stands to your side and places one hand on your upper chest. Resist as your partner gently tries to push you backward.

■ Avoid using your arms, hands or legs. Focus on the muscles of your torso.

■ Have your partner increase and decrease pressure slowly.

Partner Push #3

• STRENGTH / STABILIZATION •

RECTUS ABDOMINUS, INTERNAL AND EXTERNAL OBLIQUES, TRANSVERSE ABDOMINUS, ERECTOR SPINAE, QUADRATUS LUMBORUM

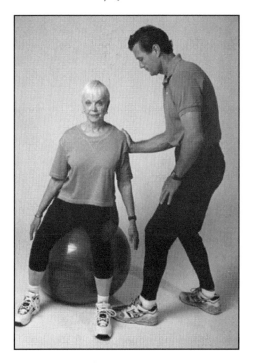

Sit on a stability ball. Have a partner stand to your right side, one hand on your upper arm. Resist as your partner gently tries to push you toward your left side.

■ Avoid using your arms, hands or legs to assist in performing this exercise.

■ Have your partner increase and decrease pressure slowly.

Battle #1

· STRENGTH / STABILIZATION ·

ERECTOR SPINAE, INTERNAL AND EXTERNAL OBLIQUES, RECTUS ABDOMINUS, TRANSVERSE
ABDOMINIUS, PECTORALIS MAJOR, SERRATUS ANTERIOR, ANTERIOR DELTOIDS

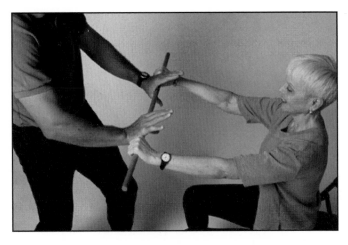

Sit holding a stick at arm's length, elbows extended. Resist as your part-ner tries to push the stick toward you.

- Have your partner give you "matching" resistance.
- Be sure to keep your elbows straight.
- Also perform with the stick held on a diagonal.
- Progress to standing or sitting on a stability ball.

Battle #2

· STRENGTH / STABILIZATION ·

ERECTOR SPINAE, INTERNAL AND EXTERNAL OBLIQUES, RECTUS ABDOMINUS,
TRANSVERSE ABDOMINUS, RHOMBOIDS, TRAPEZIUS, POSTERIOR DELTOIDS

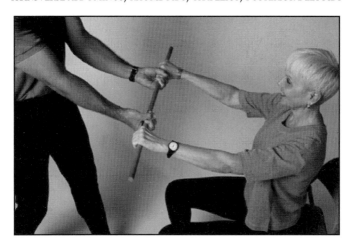

Sit holding a stick at arm's length, elbows extended. Resist as your partner tries to pull the stick away from you.

- Have your partner give you "matching" resistance.
- Be sure to keep your elbows straight.
- Also perform with the stick held on a diagonal.
- You can also do this exercise while sitting on a stability ball or
  while standing.

Buttock Squeezes

• STRENGTH •

GLUTEUS MAXIMUS

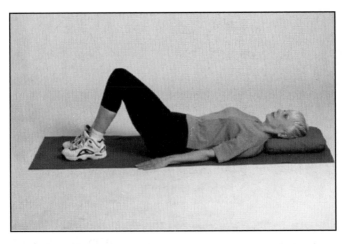

Lie on your back with your knees bent and feet together. Squeeze your buttocks together without lifting your back off the floor. Hold for 5 seconds, then release.

- Keep abdominals and thigh muscles (quadriceps and hamstrings) relaxed.
- Avoid holding your breath as you hold the contraction.
- You can also do this exercise with your feet turned out and hip distance apart.

Inner Thigh Squeezes

· STRENGTH ·

PECTINEUS, GRACILIS, ADDUCTOR MAGNUS, ADDUCTOR LONGUS, ADDUCTOR BREVIS

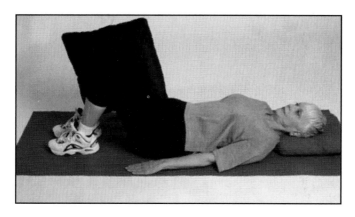

Lie on your back with the soles of your feet on the floor. Place a pillow, rolled up towel, or large ball between your knees. Squeeze the pillow using your inner thigh muscles. Hold for 5 seconds, release.

■ Keep thigh and buttock muscles (the quadriceps, hamstrings and gluteals) relaxed.

■ Breathe normally throughout.

Hip Flexion

• STRENGTH •

ILIOPSOAS, RECTUS FEMORIS

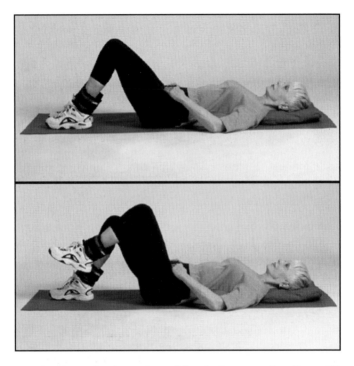

Lie on your back with the soles of both feet on the floor. Place your hands on your hip bones and engage your abdominals. Bring the right knee up 6-12 inches off the floor, then lower slowly, all the while keeping your hip bones level (do not allow the left hip bone to sink down as you lift the right leg).

- You must use your abdominal muscles to keep both hip bones aligned.
- To increase intensity, perform with a straight leg. Let the moving leg only go to the level of the opposite knee (and not any higher).
- For further challenge, add ankle weights.

Hip Rotation

· STRENGTH ·

GLUTEUS MAXIMUS, DEEP EXTERNAL ROTATORS

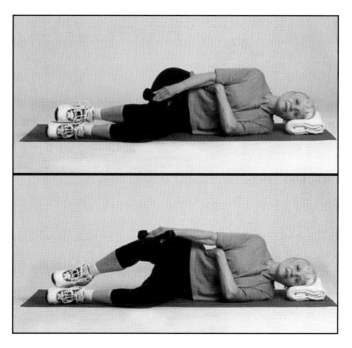

Lie on your right side. Place your head on a pillow or rolled towel. Bend both hips and knees to about 90° (as if you were sitting in a chair). Keep your feet together and lift up your left knee. Feel the work deep in your buttocks.

- Check to see that your neck and shoulders stay relaxed.
- Engage your abdominals and keep your spine lengthened.
- Increase the intensity by placing one dumbbell just above the knee.

Outer Thigh

· STRENGTH ·

GLUTEUS MEDIUS, GLUTEUS MINIMUS, TENSOR FASCIAE LATAE

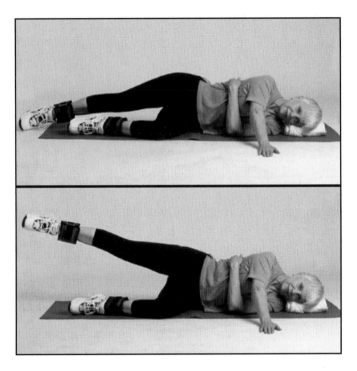

Lie on your right side with your right leg bent underneath you and your left leg straight. Your bottom and top hip should be in line. Tighten your left thigh muscles, then lift the left leg up until the leg is parallel to the floor, pause, and slowly lower.

- If you have arthritis in your hips, or are uncomfortable lying on your side, you may place a pillow under your hip bone.
- Do not "rock backwards" as you perform this exercise. You may want to turn the top foot to point toward the floor to help keep your hips stacked, one directly over the other.
- Do not let your knee bend as you lift the leg (tighten the thigh muscles).
- Maintain good body alignment while lying. Keep your abdominals in, spine lengthened, neck and shoulders relaxed.
- Add ankle weights for more challenge.

Inner Thigh

· STRENGTH ·

PECTINEUS, GRACILIS, ADDUCTOR MAGNUS, ADDUCTOR LONGUS, ADDUCTOR BREVIS

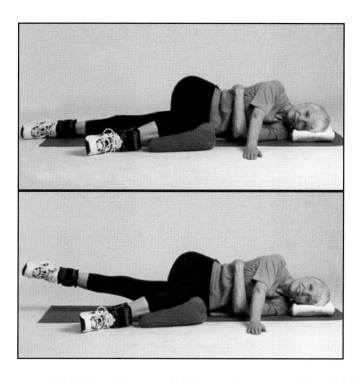

Lie on your right side with your left leg resting on a pillow in front of you. Tighten the thigh muscles of your right leg, then lift that leg up, pause, and slowly lower.

- If you have arthritis in your hips, or are uncomfortable lying on your side, place a pillow under your hip bone.
- Do not let your knee bend as you lift the leg (tighten the thigh muscles).
- Maintain good body alignment while lying. Keep your abdominals in, spine lengthened, neck and shoulders relaxed.
- Add ankle weights when you can perform 15 repetitions.

Squat with Dynaband

· STRENGTH ·

GLUTEUS MAXIMUS, QUADRICEPS

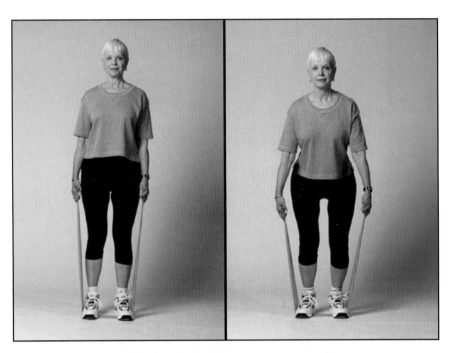

Step onto a dynaband and place your feet hip distance apart. Hold one end of the dynaband in each hand with your elbows straight. Focus straight ahead, keep a long spine, and think of pressing into your heels as you bend at the hips and knees a few inches. Return to starting position.

- The tubing should be taut throughout the movement. Shorten up on it until you feel it gives you sufficient resistance.
- Keep your elbows locked.
- The bend occurs at your hips, and not at your spine (do not do spinal flexion).
- Engage your abdominals and avoid arching your back.
- Begin by bending your knees only a few inches. You may bend further, but not past a 90° angle at the knee joint.

Step Ups

• STRENGTH / BALANCE •

GLUTEUS MAXIMUS, QUADRICEPS

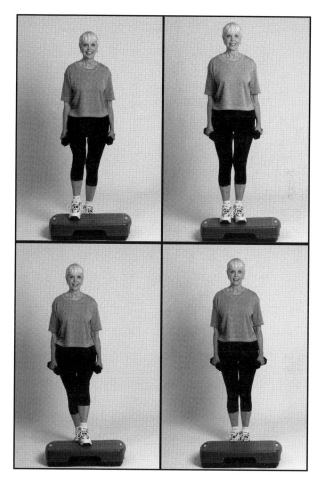

Step up onto platform with your right foot. Then bring your left foot onto the bench. Step down onto the floor with the right foot and then the left foot. Complete your repetitions beginning with the right foot before switching to the left side.

- Start with step height of 4″ or less.
- For more challenge, add one dumbbell in each hand.
- Over time, increase the height of step and the weight of the dumbbell.

Side Step Ups

• STRENGTH / BALANCE •

GLUTEUS MEDIUS, GLUTEUS MAXIMUS, QUADRICEPS, ADDUCTORS,
TENSOR FASCIAE LATAE

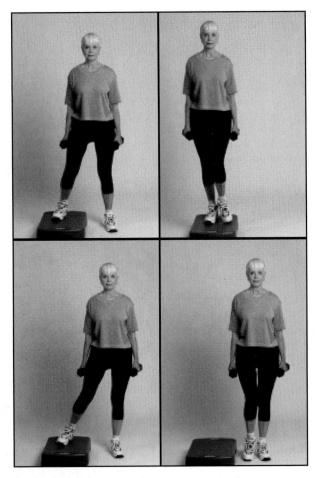

Stand with your right side to the platform. Keep your toes pointed straight ahead and step onto the platform with your right foot. Bring the left foot onto the platform. Now step back down onto the floor with your left foot, and then the right foot.

- Start with a step height of 4″ or less.
- Add one weight in each hand for added intensity.
- Over time, increase the step height and amount of weight held.

Partner Chair Sits

· STRENGTH ·

GLUTEUS MAXIMUS, QUADRICEPS

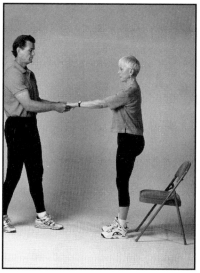 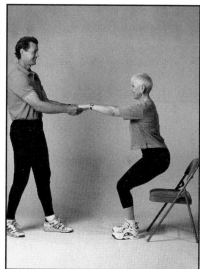

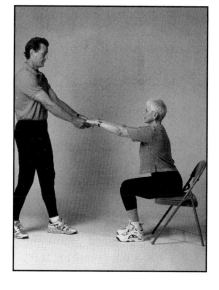

Place a stable chair behind you. Stand with your feet hip distance apart. Your partner faces you and holds onto your hands. Take 5 counts to *slowly* lower down onto the chair. Pull on your partner's hands as needed to slow your descent. Then stand up. (Have your partner help you, if needed.)

■ The key to this exercise is a very slow, controlled descent onto the chair.

■ Keep your knees over your toes as you sit and stand. In other words, avoid a "knock-kneed" position.

■ Over time, your partner should give you less assistance.

Chair Sits

· STRENGTH ·

GLUTEUS MAXIMUS, QUADRICEPS

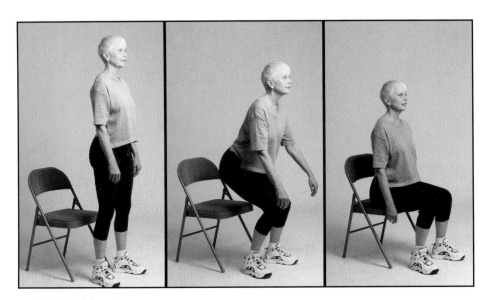

Place a stable chair behind you. Stand with feet hip distance apart. Sit down slowly onto the chair. Then stand up.

- If needed, start with a pillow placed on the chair to raise the height of the chair and make the exercise easier.
- Keep your knees over your toes as you sit and stand. Avoid a "knock-kneed" position.
- When you can easily do 15 repetitions, remove the pillow.
- Progress to holding one weight in each hand with arms at your sides.
- Progress to resting the weights on your shoulders.

Step Touches with Dynaband

· STRENGTH / BALANCE ·

GLUTEUS MEDIUS, GLUTEUS MINIMUS, TENSOR FASCIAE LATAE

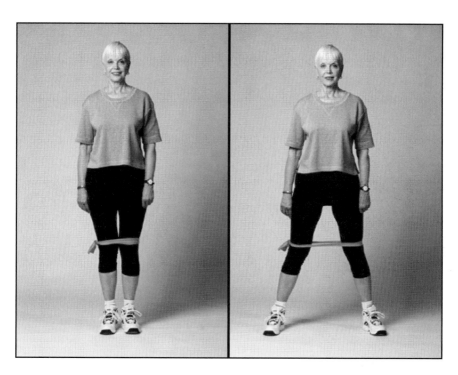

Stand with a dynaband tied just above your ankles. The tubing should be taut with your feet together. You may want to have a sturdy support for balance in front of you, or put your hand on a wall. Take a step out to the right side with your right foot. Bring your left foot in to join it. Take a step out to the left side with your left foot. Bring your right foot in to join it.

- Maintain good posture.
- Initiate the movement with the muscles along the outside of the upper thigh. Avoid using the upper body to assist with the exercise.
- To increase the intensity, take bigger steps out to the side.
- When you can easily do 20 step touches, increase to a stronger band.

Squat with Stability Ball

• STRENGTH / STABILIZATION •

GLUTEUS MAXIMUS, QUADRICEPS, HAMSTRINGS, ERECTOR SPINAE, ABDOMINALS

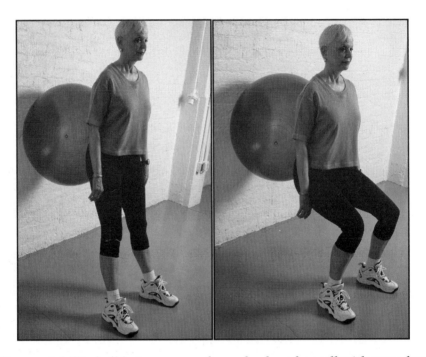

Place a stability ball between your lower back and a wall with your feet hip distance apart. Press your back into the ball and bend at the hips and knees to a squat position. The ball will roll down the wall. Slowly return to starting position so that the ball moves up the wall.

■ Do not allow your knees to extend past your toes when you squat. Your goal is to create a 90° angle between your thigh bone and your lower leg.

■ Keep your chest up throughout the movement.

■ For more challenge, use a smaller ball.

Lunges

· STRENGTH / BALANCE ·

GLUTEUS MAXIMUS, QUADRICEPS

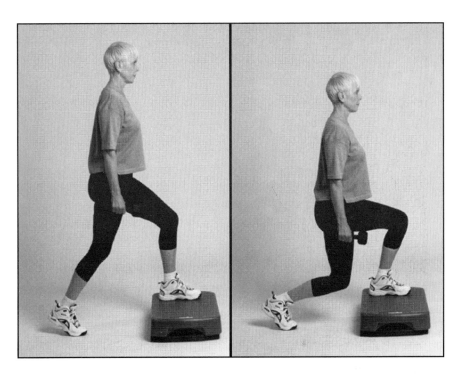

Place your right foot on a step. Come up onto the ball of the left foot so your left heel is off the floor. Bend both knees, then straighten both knees. Maintain an erect posture throughout. Do all repetitions on the right side before switching sides.

- Hold onto a support for balance, as needed.
- Avoid letting your body pitch forward. Stay centered with even weight distribution between the feet.
- Start with 3 or 4 repetitions per leg.
- Use a step with a height of 4″ or less to begin.
- To increase intensity, add one dumbbell in each hand.
- Over time, increase the height of the step as well as the weight of the dumbbell.

Jumps

· STRENGTH / POWER ·

GLUTEUS MAXIMUS, HAMSTRINGS, QUADRICEPS

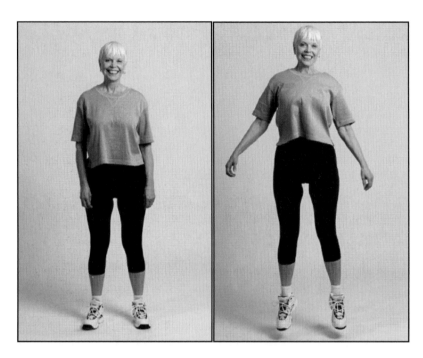

Bend your knees and then jump up so both feet momentarily leave the ground. As you touch back down onto the floor be sure to bend your knees. Your goal is to do 10 jumps in a row, rest, then repeat, until you can do 50 jumps.

■ Be sure you have physician approval before attempting this exercise. Also inquire if you can perform this exercise without shoes to give maximum stress to your hip joints.

■ This is an advanced exercise. You must have good muscle strength, especially in the torso (abdominals, erector spinae) to properly and safely execute it. (See "Abdominals" and "Spine-Lower Back" to strengthen these areas.)

Hip Rotation on Stability Ball

· FLEXIBILITY / STABILIZATION / MOBILIZATION ·

ALL THE MUSCLES SURROUNDING THE HIP JOINT, LOWER SPINE, AND ANKLES

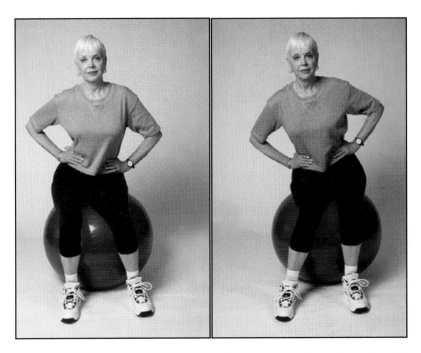

Sit on a stability ball. Move your hips slowly in a circle to the right. Then change the direction of the circle. Start with a small circle. Over time, progress to bigger and bigger circles.

Hamstring Stretch

· **FLEXIBILITY** ·

HAMSTRINGS

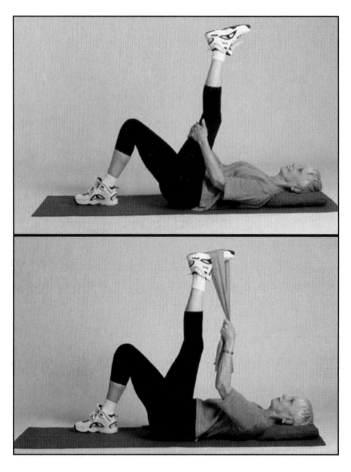

Lie on your back with the soles of both feet on the ground. Bring your right knee into your chest and place both hands under the right knee. Inhale, and as you exhale straighten the right leg as much as you can. Hold for 15 seconds while breathing normally. Repeat.

- Keep your shoulder and neck free from tension.
- A variation is placing a towel, rope, or strong dynaband under the sole of your right foot. Hold one end of whichever aid you have chosen, and then pull the leg in toward you.

Outer Thigh Stretch with Dynaband

· FLEXIBILITY ·

GLUTEUS MEDIUS, GLUTEUS MINIMUS, TENSOR FASCIAE LATAE

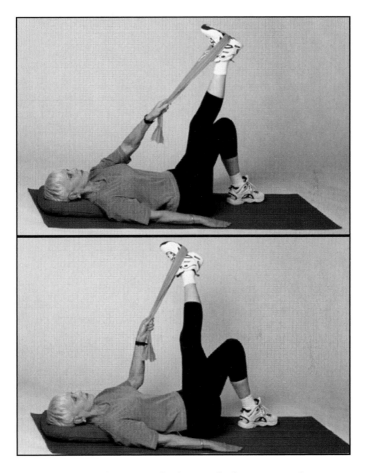

Lie on your back. Bend your right leg and place a towel, rope or strong dynaband around the sole of the right foot, holding *both* ends in your *left* hand. Straighten your right leg as much as you can. Then pull with your left hand to bring the right leg over toward the *left* side.

- Keep your neck and shoulder muscles relaxed.
- You may let your torso slightly twist toward the left to increase the stretch.

Inner Thigh Stretch with Dynaband

• FLEXIBILITY •

PECTINEUS, GRACILIS, ADDUCTOR MAGNUS, ADDUCTOR LONGUS, ADDUCTOR BREVIS

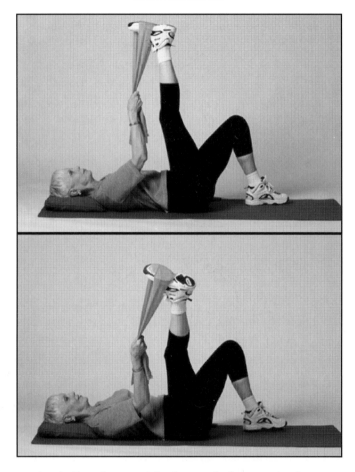

Lie on your back. Bend your right leg and place a towel, rope or strong dynaband around the sole of the right foot. Hold *both* ends of the towel in your *right* hand. Straighten the leg as much as you can. Then pull with your right hand to bring the leg over toward the *right* side.

■ Engage your abdominals to keep your hip bones level.
■ Do not overdo this stretch. You should feel a gentle stretch in your inner thigh but no pain.

Hip Flexor Stretch

· FLEXIBILITY ·

ILIOPSOAS, RECTUS FEMORIS

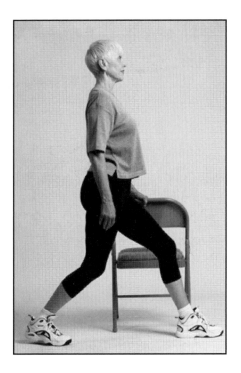

Stand in a staggered lunge position with your right foot forward. Hold onto a support for balance, if needed. Bend both knees slightly. Gently lift your torso so that you lean back slightly or just until you feel a stretch in the front of left hip and upper thigh.

■ Do not let the front knee bend beyond the toes of the front foot.
■ To increase the stretch, take the front foot further forward.

Towel Wrings

· STRENGTH ·

FLEXOR CARPI RADIALIS, PALMARIS LONGUS, FLEXOR CARPI ULNARIS, EXTENSOR CARPI ULNARIS, EXTENSOR CARPI RADIALIS BREVIS, EXTENSOR CARPI RADIALIS LONGUS, FLEXOR DIGITORUM SUPERFICIALIS, FLEXOR DIGITORUM PROFUNDUS, FLEXOR POLLICIS LONGUS

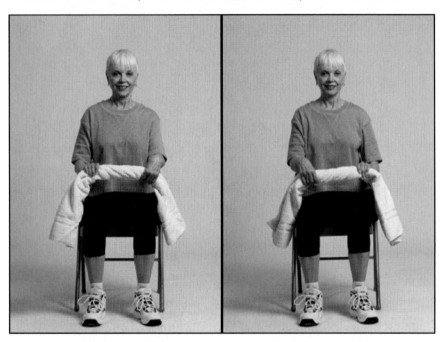

Hold a towel with your elbows bent and next to your sides. Try to "wring" out a towel so that one wrist extends as the other wrist flexes. Then reverse.

- Don't grip too tightly.
- Focus on the wrist muscles doing the work, not the finger muscles.

Ball Squeezes

• STRENGTH •

FLEXOR DIGITORUM SUPERFICIALIS, FLEXOR DIGITORUM PROFUNDUS,
FLEXOR POLLICIS LONGUS

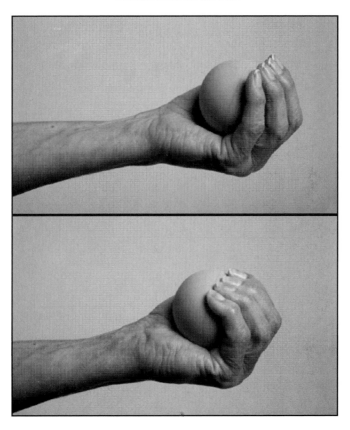

Rest your left forearm on your lap (or on a table). Hold a ball in your left hand with your palm up. Keep the back of the hand touching your lap (or table) as you squeeze the ball with your fingers. Hold for 3 seconds.

- Maintain a neutral wrist. Do not let the wrist bend backwards or forwards.
- Keep your 3rd finger in line with the middle of your wrist . This will avoid ulnar or radial deviation, a misalignment that can put stress on your wrist joint.

79

Wrist Flexion

· STRENGTH ·

FLEXOR CARPI RADIALIS, PALMARIS LONGUS, FLEXOR CARPI ULNARIS, FLEXOR DIGITORUM
SUPERFICIALIS, FLEXOR DIGITORUM PROFUNDUS, FLEXOR POLLICIS LONGUS

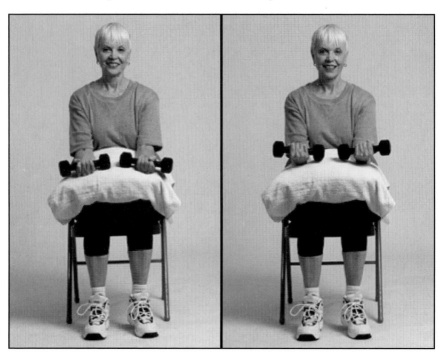

Rest your forearms on your lap (or on a table) with one dumbbell in
each hand, palms facing up. Bend at the wrists so your palms move
toward the forearms. Pause, then slowly return to starting position.

- Avoid holding the dumbbells too tightly.
- Keep your 3rd finger directly in line with the middle of your
  wrist.

Wrist Extension

• STRENGTH •

EXTENSOR CARPI ULNARIS, EXTENSOR CARPI RADIALIS BREVIS, EXTENSOR CARPI RADIALIS LONGUS, EXTENSOR DIGITORUM, EXTENSOR POLLICIS LONGUS

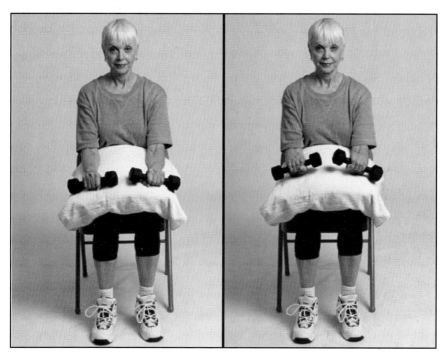

Rest your forearms on your lap (or on a table) with one dumbbell in each hand, palms facing down. Bend at the wrists so the back of your hands move toward your forearms. Pause, return to starting position.

- Avoid holding the dumbbells too tightly.
- Keep your 3rd finger directly in line with the middle of your wrist.

Swimming Strokes

• FLEXIBILITY / MOBILIZATION •

ALL THE MUSCLES OF THE SHOULDER JOINT AND SCAPULA

CRAWL STROKE

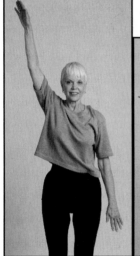 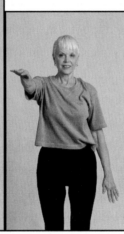

Stand with knees slightly bent, abdominals engaged, head up. Do the crawl stroke with the right arm, and with the left arm. Then do the back stroke with the right and left arms. Next do the breast stroke using both arms simultaneously. Finally, do the butterfly stroke using both arms together.

■ Stay in a pain free range of motion. You may need to begin with very small movements and, over time, gradually make the strokes bigger.

■ Keep both hip bones facing forward throughout all the exercises.

BACK STROKE

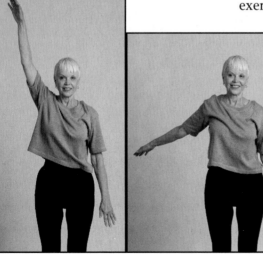

■ After completing the 4 strokes, perform the back stroke letting your head watch your arm as it reaches as far back as you can. In this instance, your hips will move and your torso will rotate.

BREAST STROKE

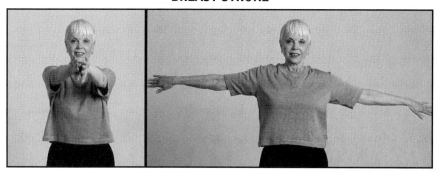

BUTTERFLY STROKE

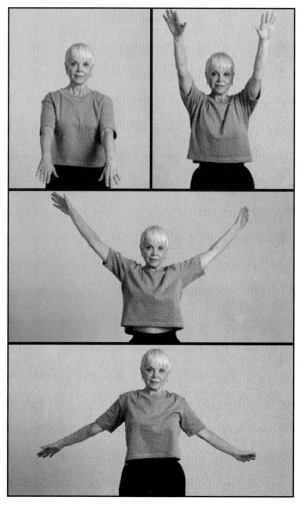

Angel Arms

· STRENGTH / FLEXIBILITY ·

PECTORALIS MAJOR, SERRATUS ANTERIOR, DELTOIDS, SUPRASPINATUS

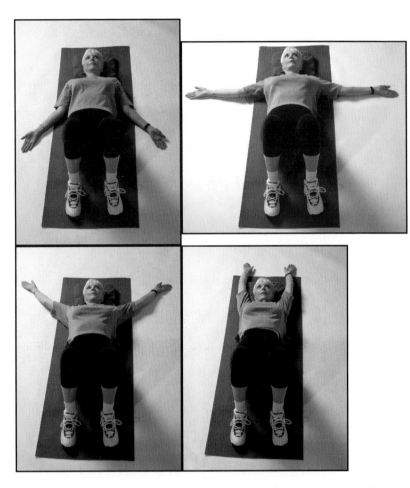

Lie on your back with your arms down by your side, palms up. Now, bring your arms 1" off the floor. Keep your elbows straight as you bring your arms away from your sides in an arc until they are overhead. Return to starting position using the same pattern. Think of making angels in the snow.

Protraction with Dynaband

· STRENGTH ·

SERRRATUS ANTERIOR

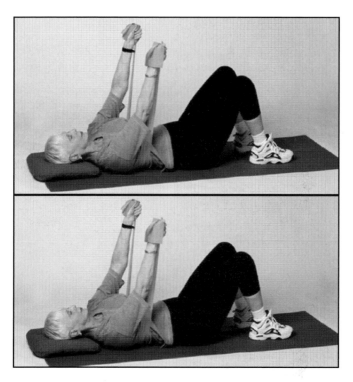

Lie on your back with a dynaband around your back and just under your armpits. Hold one end of the tubing in each hand, palms facing each other, and press straight up. This is the starting position. Now, keep the elbows straight as you lift your shoulder blades off the floor and feel them move apart from one another (protraction). Pause, lower slowly with the elbows remaining straight, and bring your shoulder blades together (retraction).

■ This is an important exercise to do if you have any "winging" of your scapula, that is, if your shoulder blades are not resting flat against your spine.

■ Your head remains on the floor.

■ Do not raise your shoulders towards your ears. Shoulders stay relaxed.

■ The elbows do not bend at all. If you do so, you will be using other muscles to perform this exercise.

Chest Press with Dynaband

• STRENGTH •

PECTORALIS MAJOR, SERRATUS ANTERIOR, ANTERIOR DELTOIDS, TRICEPS

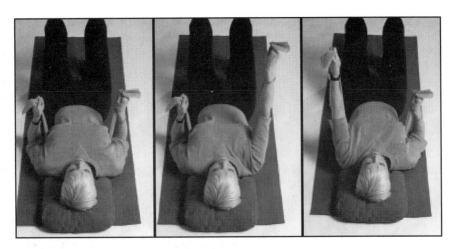

Lie on the floor with a dynaband around your back just below the armpits. Hold one end of the tubing in each hand, elbows bent, palms facing each other. Press the right arm straight up until the elbow completely straightens and you feel your right shoulder blade coming off the floor. Pause, return slowly to starting position.

■ Push up with the band so your arm is over your mid chest and *not* over your neck.

■ Lengthen or shorten the tubing, or change to a heavier or lighter tubing, to get the correct amount of resistance to challenge you.

■ Keep a neutral wrist throughout movement. Do not allow your wrist to bend backwards.

■ The shoulders and neck remain relaxed.

Wall Push Up

· STRENGTH ·

PECTORALIS MAJOR, SERRATUS ANTERIOR, ANTERIOR DELTOIDS, TRICEPS;
ALSO WRIST STRENGTHENER*

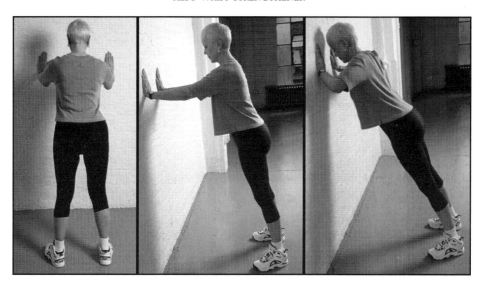

Stand facing a wall at a distance. Reach out to place your palms on the wall at a level slightly below your shoulders. Your elbows are extended and you should feel that you need to stretch to touch the wall. (This brings your shoulder blades apart.) Now, bend your elbows so that they move toward the floor as your body moves toward the wall. Pause, then straighten elbows.

■ Do not do this exercise if you feel any pain or discomfort in your wrist.

■ Keep your head in one position throughout the movement; do not allow it to either drop or to move forward.

■ The abdominals should be held in tightly so that your body does not sag.

■ For added challenge, have a partner place a hand over your mid back and give you gentle resistance as you push away from the wall.

Shoulder Rotation with Dynaband

· STRENGTH / POSTURE ·

POSTERIOR DELTOIDS, INFRASPINATUS, TERES MINOR

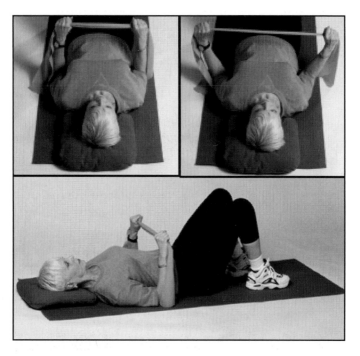

Lie on your back. Hold each end of a dynaband and bend your elbows to form a 90° angle. Keep the back of your arms on the floor as you gently pull the dynaband apart. Pause, return to starting position. Adjust the length of the dynaband to increase or decrease the tension.

- Be sure you perform this exercise with a neutral wrist.
- Do not allow the elbows to move away from your sides as they will have a tendency to do.
- Keep tension in the dynaband. Do not allow it to snap back.
- Performed correctly, you will feel this exercise in your shoulder joint.

Press Up

· **STRENGTH** ·

PECTORALIS MAJOR, SERRATUS ANTERIOR, DELTOIDS, TRICEPS

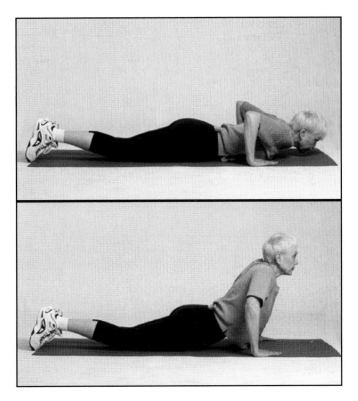

Lie on your stomach with your palms on the floor under your armpits, elbows in towards your sides, and abdominals engaged. Push up, straighten your elbows as much as possible, and let the shoulder blades move apart. This brings your upper body off the floor but leaves your hips and thighs on the floor. Pause, lower slowly.

- Your goal is to maintain a straight line from your head to your hips. Keep your abdominals tight and avoid any arch or sagging in your back.
- Your head stays in line with your spine. Do not let it to either drop down or jerk back to help with the lift.

Full Body Hold

• STRENGTH / STABILIZATION •

PECTORALIS MAJOR, SERRATUS ANTERIOR, DELTOIDS,
TRICEPS AND MOST OF THE MUSCLES OF THE LOWER BODY

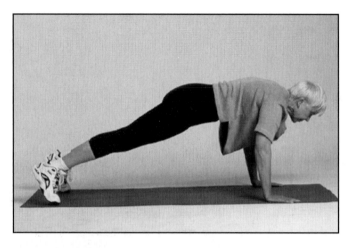

Begin on your hands and toes (the standard push up position). Your shoulders blades should be far apart, abdominals tight, and head in line with your spine. Hold the position for 10 seconds.

- Keep abdominals tight. Do not sag in the middle.
- To increase intensity, hold the position for a longer period of time.

Chest Stretch

· FLEXIBILITY ·

PECTORALIS MAJOR, PECTORALIS MINOR, ANTERIOR DELTOIDS

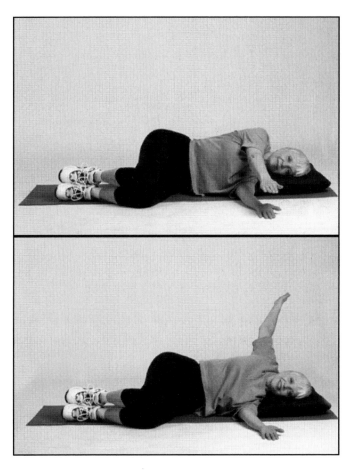

Lie on your right side with both knees bent (as if you were sitting in a chair). Keep your chest up and your spine lengthened and bring both arms straight out in front so that your left arm is just above your right arm. Lift your left arm up in an arc and press it back gently until you feel a stretch in your left chest area. You may let your body twist slightly to the left in concert with the arm movement to increase the stretch.

Full Body Stretch

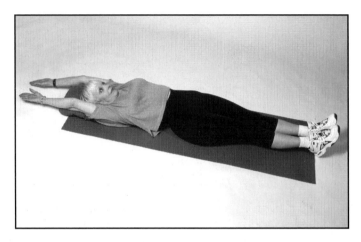

Lie on your back with your legs extended. Reach both arms overhead and let them gently drop behind your head as far as you can. Take a deep breath, then exhale and bring your arms back down to your sides.

- You may not be able to get your arms close to the floor at all. Just relax into the stretch at whatever point you are.
- Imagine that someone is pulling at your wrists at the same time that someone else is pulling at your ankles, so that you feel your whole body lengthening.

Kegels

· STRENGTH ·

PELVIC FLOOR MUSCLES AND LOWER FIBERS OF RECTUS ABDOMINUS

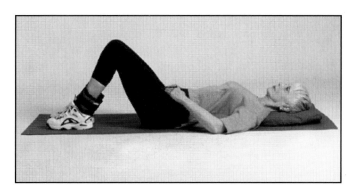

Kegels strengthen the muscles that support many of the internal organs, such as the bladder. You can practice locating these muscles by stopping the flow of urine a few times. Once you know how to engage them, do this exercise while lying down. Think of the pelvic floor as an elevator. Contract the pelvic floor muscles (perform a Kegel) and see the pelvic floor go up a flight on the elevator. Contract them even more strongly and go up another flight. Still without letting go, contract them even stronger yet and go up another flight. Hold for a moment, then release slowly, one floor at a time. At the bottom, do a gentle "push" outwards.

- In order for this exercise to be effective, you must *not* engage your abdominals, buttocks or thighs; these need to stay relaxed.
- For more challenge, you can add more "flights" on your elevator.
- Progress to performing this exercise while standing.

In and Up

• STRENGTH •

TRANSVERSE ABDOMINUS, RECTUS ABDOMINUS,
INTERNAL AND EXTERNAL OBLIQUES

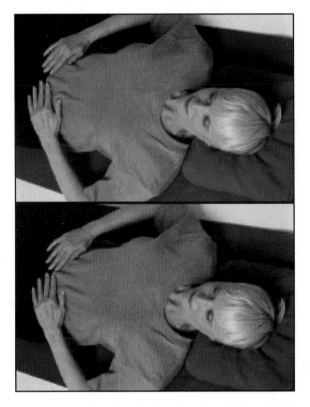

Place your hands on either side of your stomach at the level of your belly button. Now think of narrowing your waist as you contract your abdominal muscles. You should see your hands move slightly closer to one another. Then think of pulling your belly button down in the direction of your spine. Next think of pulling your belly button up towards your ribcage. Hold for a count of three, then release.

- You should not see your chest expand.
- Do not flatten your spine, or press down with your lower back.
- Be sure not to tuck your pelvis under. Your buttock muscles remain relaxed and do not rise up off the floor.
- No "bones" should move (keep the chest and pelvis out of the exercise). Isolate the abdominal muscles.

Lean Back

· STRENGTH ·

RECTUS ABDOMINUS

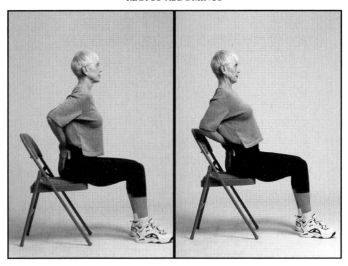

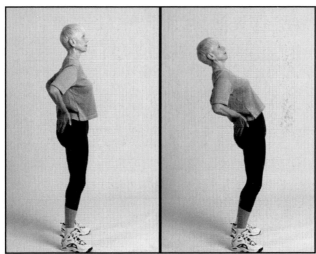

Sit on the forward edge of a chair. Place your hands behind you along your lower back. Now lean backwards slowly, pause, then return to an upright position.

- Do not do this exercise if it makes you dizzy.
- You may progress to performing this exercise while standing.

Belly Button

· **STRENGTH** ·

RECTUS ABDOMINUS, INTERNAL AND EXTERNAL OBLIQUES,
TRANSVERSE ABDOMINUS

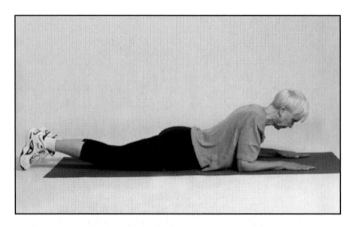

Lie on your stomach with your hands and elbows on the floor and your head up in alignment with your spine. Contract your abdominals so that you pull your belly button off the floor. Hold, then release slowly.

■ Each time try to pull your belly button up even higher off the floor so that you engage your abdominals more deeply with each lift.
■ Continue to breathe normally throughout.

Knee Twist

• STRENGTH •

RECTUS ABDOMINUS, INTERNAL AND EXTERNAL OBLIQUES, ERECTOR SPINAE

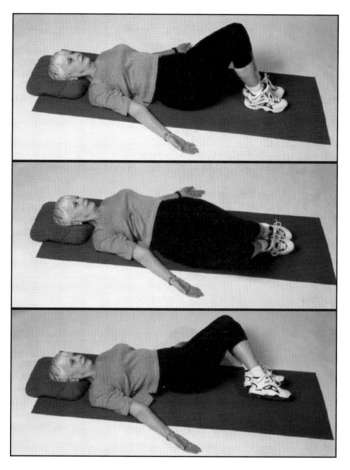

Lie on your back with your arms out to the side. Your feet are together on the floor with your knees bent. Take four counts to slowly lower both knees towards the right side, but do not let them touch the floor. Pause, then take four counts to slowly return to starting position. Pause, then slowly lower both knees to the left side.

- Begin by moving just a few inches to each side.
- Focus on the abdominal muscles controlling the movement and not the muscles in your hips or legs.

97

Side to Side

• STRENGTH •

RECTUS ABDOMINUS, INTERNAL AND EXTERNAL OBLIQUES,
ERECTOR SPINAE

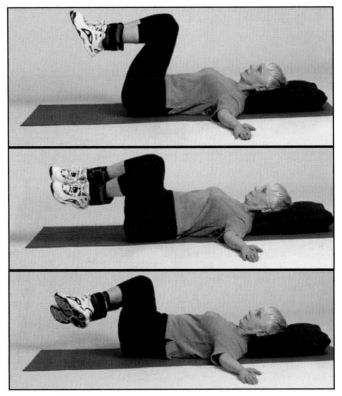

Lie on your back. Lift your right knee up and then your left knee. Take 4 counts to slowly lower both knees toward the right side. Pause, then take 4 counts to slowly return knees back to the middle. Pause, then slowly lower both knees toward the left side.

- Begin by moving just a few inches to each side.
- You need not lower the knees all the way to the floor. Just go as far as is comfortable.
- Focus on the abdominal muscles performing the movement, and not your leg muscles.
- Increase intensity by adding ankle weights.
- A very advanced progression is keeping the legs straight so that the exercise looks like "windshield wipers."

Reverse Curl

· **STRENGTH** ·

RECTUS ABDOMINUS

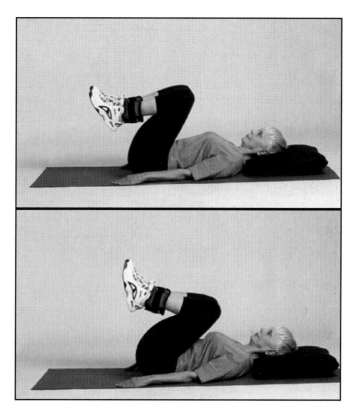

Lie on your back. Lift your right knee up and then your left knee. This is the beginning position for the exercise. Use the abdominal muscles to bring your pubic bone toward your ribcage. Pause, release just a little, and then repeat the movement. Keep the work in the abdominal muscles and avoid using momentum.

- After completing the repetitions for this exercise, place your right foot on the floor followed by your left foot. (This reduces stress to the lower back.)
- The range of motion is very small; about 6 inches up and 6 inches down.
- To increase intensity, add ankle weights.

Reverse Curl with Stability Ball

· STRENGTH ·

RECTUS ABDOMINUS

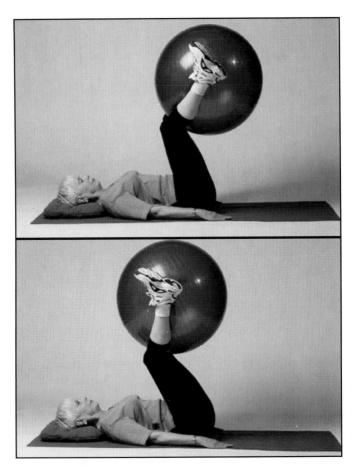

Lie on your back. Place a stability ball between your feet and lower legs with your knees bent. Contract the abdominal muscles to bring your pubic bone closer to your ribcage (this brings the legs in closer to your chest). Pause, then release a few inches down (to keep tension in the abdominals) and repeat movement.

- The range of movement is very small; about 6 inches up and 6 inches down.
- This is a real tough one. Kudos to you if you can do it!

Ankle Circles

· FLEXIBILITY ·

ALL THE MUSCLES OF THE ANKLE JOINT

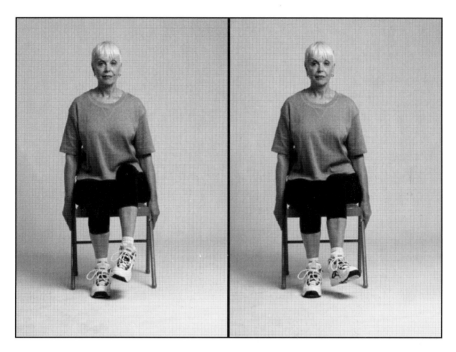

Bring your right knee up toward your chest. (You can be seated or lying on your back.) Circle the ankle to the right. Complete all repetitions. Then circle to the left.

- Make the circle as large as possible and perform the movement slowly.
- Only your foot should be moving. Avoid any movement at the knee or lower leg.
- A variation is performing a "figure eight" in each direction.

Toe Taps

· STRENGTH ·

ANTERIOR TIBIALIS

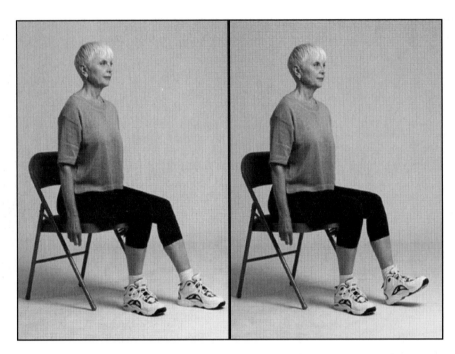

Sit in a chair with both feet flat on the floor and toes pointing straight ahead. Lift your left foot up toward your shin as high as possible while keeping your heel on the floor. Lower slowly.

- You should feel the work being done by the muscles located on the front of your shin. If you do not, extend the left leg out in front a little more (further away from you).
- For added intensity, place an ankle weight over the top of the foot.

Calf Raises

· STRENGTH / STRETCH ·

GASTROCNEMIUS, SOLEUS

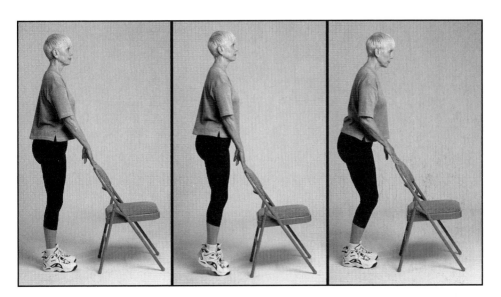

Stand holding onto a sturdy object for support, if needed. Rise up onto your toes as high as possible. Pause, then slowly lower down. Now gently bend the knees so that you feel a stretch in your calf muscles. Hold, then return to starting position.

■ Progress to performing this exercise without holding on.
■ Add one dumbbell in each hand when you can perform the exercise without support.
■ Continue to increase the weight of the dumbbells over time.

Heel Walks

• STRENGTH / BALANCE •

ANTERIOR TIBIALIS

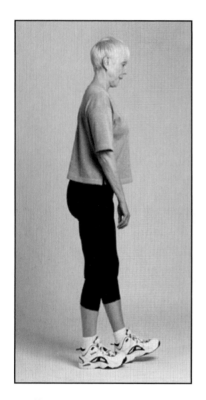
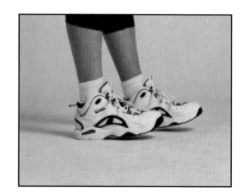

Walk on your heels. Keep the balls of the foot lifted up off the floor. Keep your body as erect as you can.

- Begin along a wall so you can place one hand on the wall for balance as needed.
- Keep your chest up. Avoid bending from the waist.

Toe Walks

· STRENGTH / BALANCE ·

GASTROCNEMIUS, SOLEUS

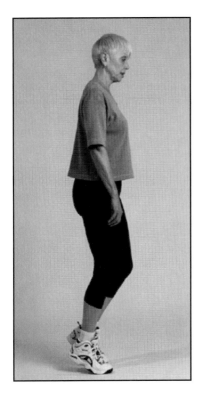

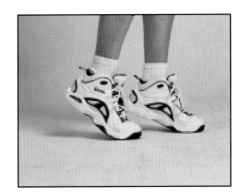

Walk on your toes. Keep your body erect.

- Begin along a wall so you can place one hand on the wall for balance as needed.
- Keep your chest up and avoid bending from the waist.

Ankle Bend with Dynaband

• STRENGTH / BALANCE •

ANTERIOR TIBIALIS

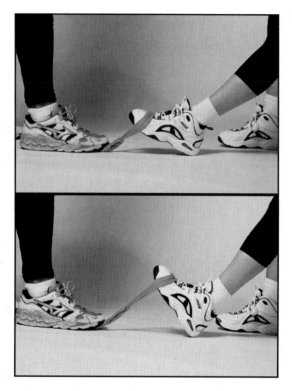

Place a dynaband over the top of one foot and secure the two ends by tying it to a secure object or having someone step on it. (You can be seated or standing.) Keep your heel on the floor and lift up your foot. Pause, lower slowly.

■ You should feel this exercise work the muscle along the front of your shin bone (the anterior tibialis). This is an important muscle to keep strong in order to prevent falling.

■ Shorten or lengthen the band to get the right challenge for you. Over time, progress to a heavier dynaband.

Grapevine

• BALANCE / COORDINATION •

THE WHOLE BODY

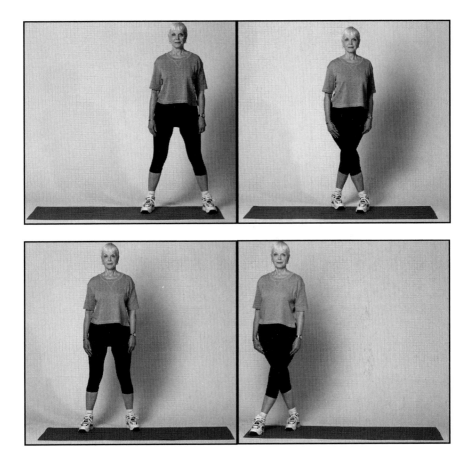

Stand so that you have space to move sideways to the right. Take a step out to the side with the right foot. Then cross the left foot over the right. Take a step out to the side with the right foot again. Then cross the left foot behind the right foot. Keep repeating until you run out of space. Then begin with the left foot stepping out to the side. Your goal is to progressively increase the speed.

107

Walk Around

• BALANCE / COORDINATION •

THE WHOLE BODY

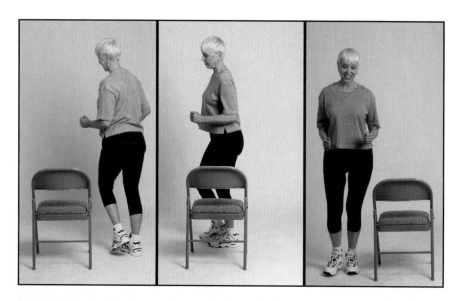

Place a chair, bench, or large object on the floor with space to walk around it on all sides. Walk around the object clockwise as fast as you can. Turn and walk counterclockwise as fast as you can. Pause so you don't get dizzy, then repeat.

One Leg Stand

· STRENGTH / BALANCE ·

THE WHOLE BODY

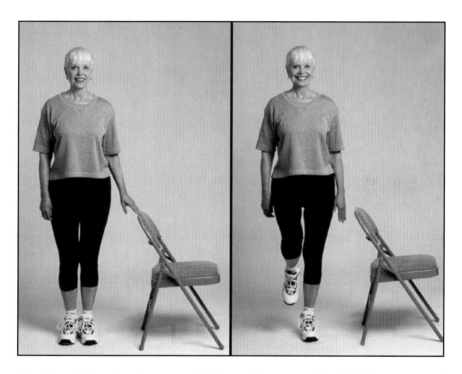

Stand next to a sturdy support. Lift one leg up and hold it for a count of 10. Change legs. Your goal is to do this exercise without having to hold on to anything for balance. When you need more of a challenge, do the exercise with your eyes closed.

One Leg Stand with Knee Bend

• STRENGTH / BALANCE •

THE WHOLE BODY

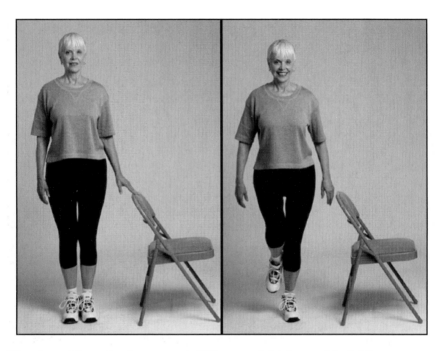

Stand next to a sturdy support. Lift your right leg and hold it up as you bend and straighten the left leg 10 times. Your goal is to do this exercise without having to hold on to anything for balance.

One Leg Stand with Arm Swing

• STRENGTH / BALANCE •

THE WHOLE BODY

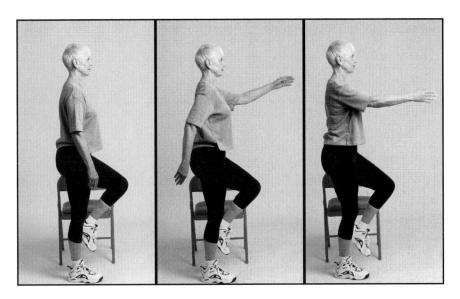

Stand next to a sturdy support. Lift your right leg and hold the leg up as you swing your arms forward and back in opposition (right arm forward with left arm backward). Keep swinging the arms for a count of 10. Change legs.

- Begin lifting your foot off the floor one or two inches and swinging your arms only slightly.
- Gradually lift your foot higher and increase the movement of the arms.
- Keep your chest up. Avoid bending from the waist.
- When you're ready for more challenge, try it with your eyes closed.

Ball Catch

• BALANCE / COORDINATION •

THE WHOLE BODY

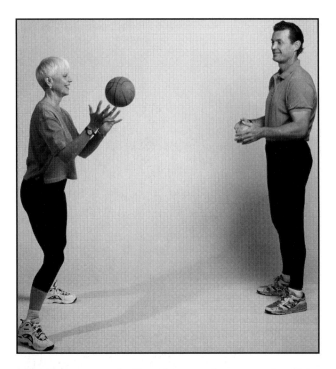

Have a partner throw you a ball so that you have to take a big step to the right or to the left to catch it. A variation is to *stand on one foot*, and then have your partner throw the ball to you so you have to slightly lean over to one side to catch it.

Calf Stretch with Dynaband

· STRETCH ·

GASTROCNEMIUS

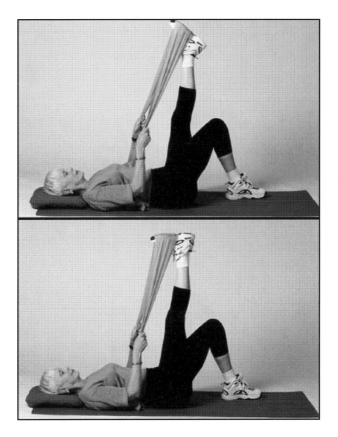

Lie on your back and place a dynaband around the sole of your right foot. Hold one end of the dynaband in each hand. Straighten your right leg (keep a very slight bend in the knee). Flex your right foot so your toes move toward your shin. Pull on the dynaband to assist you with the stretch. Pause, then release gently.

- Keep your head down.
- Your neck and shoulders stay relaxed.
- Remember to keep breathing.

Deep Calf Stretch with Dynaband

· STRETCH ·

SOLEUS

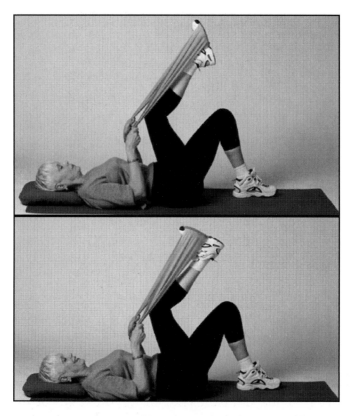

Lie on your back with a dynaband around the sole of your right foot. Hold one end of the dynaband in each hand. Lift up your right leg and behind the knee. Bring the toes of your right foot toward your shin. Pull on the dynaband to assist you with the stretch. Pause, then release gently.

- Keep your head down.
- Avoid tension in your neck and shoulders.
- Breathe normally.

Chest

· MOBILIZATION ·

INTERCOSTALS, DIAPHRAGM

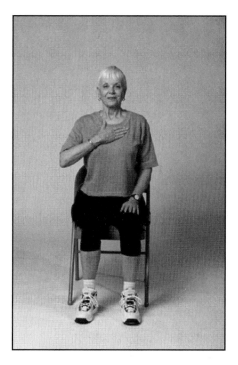

Place one hand on the top of your chest, just below your collar bone. Inhale as deeply as you can and direct your breath into your hand. Feel the air go only under your hand (and not anywhere else in your body). Pause, then exhale slowly so that you "push" all the air out. Relax all the other muscles of your body and avoid lifting your shoulders. Do 2 times.

- You may begin with 5 counts to inhale, and 5 counts to exhale. Gradually, increase to 10 counts.
- Over time, try to increase how deeply you inhale.

Diaphragm

· MOBILIZATION ·

INTERCOSTALS, DIAPHRAGM

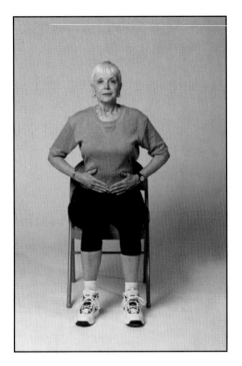

Place one hand over your stomach at the level of your belly button. Inhale as deeply as you can and direct your breath into your hand. See your hand move as the air enters your stomach. Your chest should not rise. Pause, then exhale slowly so that you "push" all the air out. Relax all the other muscles of your body and avoid lifting your shoulders. Do 2 times.

- Start with 5 counts to inhale and 5 counts to exhale. Over time, progress to breathing in for 10 counts, and breathing out for 10 counts.
- Your goal is to increase the depth of your inhalation.

Ribcage

• MOBILIZATION •

INTERCOSTALS, DIAPHRAGM

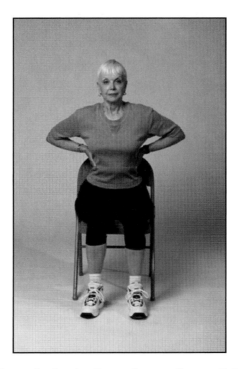

Place both hands on the back of your lower ribcage. Inhale as deeply as you can and direct your breath into your hands. Feel the air going into the area your hands are, and not anywhere else (neither your chest nor your abdomen should rise). Pause, then exhale slowly so that you "push" all the air out. Relax all the other muscles of your body and avoid lifting your shoulders. Do 2 times.

- When you breathe in you should feel the air pushing your hands apart.
- Progress to breathing in for 10 counts, and breathing out for 10 counts.
- Over time try to increase the amount of air you take in with each breath.

117

Three Dimensional

· MOBILIZATION ·

INTERCOSTALS, DIAPHRAGM

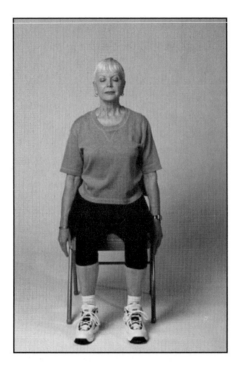

Inhale as deeply as you can, letting the breath fill your upper chest, abdomen and back of your ribcage. Pause, then exhale slowly. Relax all the other muscles of your body and avoid lifting your shoulders.

- Progress to breathing in for 10 counts, and breathing out for 10 counts.
- Feel your entire torso expand with your inhalation.
- Your goal is to increase the amount of air you take in with each breath.

CHAPTER NINE

Focus on how good you feel *after* exercise—more energy, improved mood, a sense of accomplishment, and empowerment.

A Good Time to Start

HE PERSON WHO INVENTS a pill to get us to do just what we should be doing at any given moment would undoubtedly become the richest, and most famous, person in the world. While we await that miracle we are faced with the challenge of integrating exercise into our everyday lives regardless of our motivation, time constraints, or energy level. The benefits of exercise, unfortunately, are short-lasting. And the older we get, the faster those benefits evaporate.

For exercise to be effective, we're faced with a lifetime commitment. So how do we make exercise an integral part of our lives?

- **Just do it**. Nike got it right. There's no right time to start exercise. Life's responsibilities will always intrude. We'll always be busy at work, or have our family to take care of, or major commitments to honor, or just not have all the pieces in our fabric of life aligned just so as to remove all hindrances. If you wait for the perfect time to start, you may find that day just never comes.

- **Savor your accomplishment**. Give yourself a pat on the back for your effort when the exercise session is over. Even if it's a half-hearted workout, you did it! Some days 50% is all you have to give.

- **Make it a habit**. Try to schedule exercise at the same time each day. The positive effects of exercise are only maintained as long as the exercise is continued. It cannot be stored up and "saved for a rainy day."

- **Prompts**. Writing "exercise, 6 P.M." in your daily appointment book, keeping an exercise journal or log, even stashing your exercise paraphernalia in a visible place, can all be effective visual motivators.

- **Don't be hard on yourself**. If you can't exercise, for whatever reason, for a day, a week, or a month, so be it. Be secure in the knowledge that you can, and will, get back on the exercise wagon. Reminding yourself how strong and energetic you felt when you were exercising can motivate you to begin again.

CHAPTER TEN

Programs

OSTEOPOROSIS · PROGRAM 1

EQUIPMENT: Pillow, towel
EXERCISE POSITIONS: Lying, seated
PROGRESSION: Add an additional set. Use ankle weights for exercises indicated with
                    asterisk (*). Proceed to Program 2.

NECK

Resisted Neck #1 .... 3 reps
Resisted Neck #2 .... 3 reps
Resisted Neck #3 .... 3 reps, do both sides

SPINE: UPPER/MID BACK

Retraction .... 12 reps
Bent Arm Retraction .... 12 reps

SPINE: LOWER BACK

Spine Press .... 4 reps
Modified Trunk Lift .... 4 reps
Knee to Chest .... hold 15 secs, each leg, do twice

TORSO STABILIZATION

Bridge .... 8 reps

HIP

Buttock Squeezes .... 8 reps
Inner Thigh Squeezes .... 8 reps
Hip Flexion * .... 8 reps, each leg
Hip Rotation * .... 8 reps, each leg

WRIST

Towel Wrings .... 8 times, switching directions

CHEST-ARMS

Angel Arms .... 8 times
Chest Stretch .... hold 15 secs, each side, do twice

ABDOMINALS

Kegels .... 8 reps
In and Up .... 8 reps
Knee Twist .... 8 times, each direction

BALANCE

Ankle Circles .... 8 times each direction
Toe Taps .... 8 reps, each foot

BREATHING

Chest .... do 2 times
Ribcage .... do 2 times
Diaphragm .... do 2 times

OSTEOPOROSIS · PROGRAM 2

EQUIPMENT NEEDED: Dynaband, small ball, chair, wall
EXERCISE POSITIONS: Lying, seated, standing, walking
PROGRESSION: Add an additional set. Change to a heavier dynaband. Proceed to Program 3 or 4.

NECK

Resisted Neck #1 .... 5 reps
Resisted Neck #2 .... 5 reps
Resisted Neck #3 .... 5 reps, do both sides

SPINE: UPPER/MID BACK

Reverse Fly *with dynaband* .... 8 reps, each arm

SPINE: LOWER BACK

Walking with Rotation .... 10 walks forward

TORSO STABILIZATION

One-Legged Bridge .... 8 reps, each leg

HIP

Squat *with dynaband* .... 8 reps
Outer Thigh .... 8 reps
Hip Flexor Stretch .... hold 15 secs, each leg

WRIST

Ball Squeezes .... 8 reps, each hand

CHEST-ARMS

Swimming Strokes .... 8 reps, each stroke
Wall Push Up .... 8 reps
Full Body Stretch .... hold 15 secs

ABDOMINALS

In and Up .... 8 reps
Lean Back .... 8 reps
Knee Twist .... 8 reps right and left

BALANCE

Grapevine .... 12 steps, each direction
Walk Around .... 2 times, each direction
Ankle Bend *with dynaband* .... 8 reps, each foot
Calf Stretch *with dynaband* .... hold 15 secs, each leg, do twice
Deep Calf Stretch *with dynaband* .... hold 15 secs, each leg, do twice

BREATHING

Chest .... do 2 times
Ribcage .... do 2 times
Diaphragm .... do 2 times
Three Dimensional .... do 2 times

OSTEOPENIA · PROGRAM 3

EQUIPMENT NEEDED: Dynaband, step, chair, small ball, towel
EXERCISE POSITIONS: Lying, seated, standing, walking, stepping up and down
PROGRESSION: Use stronger dynaband, or add ankle weights and dumbbells for
                      exercises indicated with asterisk (*). Proceed to Program 4.

NECK

Head Lift Back .... 8 reps
Head Lift Side .... 8 reps, do both sides

SPINE: UPPER/MID BACK

Row *with dynaband* .... 8 reps, 2 sets

SPINE: LOWER BACK

Hip Walks .... 8 walks forward, 8 back
Four Point Arm and Leg Raise* .... switch arms and legs 8 times

TORSO STABILIZATION

Pelvic Stabilization .... lift right and left foot up 8 times

HIP

Step Ups* .... 8 step ups, each leg
Side Step Ups* .... 8 step ups, each leg
Chair Sits* .... 8 reps

WRIST

Ball Squeezes .... 8 reps, 2 sets, each hand

CHEST & ARMS

Shoulder Rotation *with dynaband* .... 8 reps, each arm
Protraction *with dynaband* .... 8 reps
Chest Press *with dynaband* .... 8 reps
Chest Stretch .... hold 15 secs, each side

ABDOMINALS

Reverse Curl* .... 10 reps
Side to Side* .... 10 times right and left

BALANCE

Heel Walks .... forward 10 steps, backward 10 steps
Toe Walks .... forward 10 steps, backward 10 stes
One Leg Stand .... hold 10 secs, 2 sets, each leg

BREATHING

Chest .... do 2 times
Ribcage .... do 2 times
Diaphragm .... do 2 times
Three Dimensional .... do 2 times

OSTEOPENIA · PROGRAM 4

EQUIPMENT NEEDED: Dumbbells, chair, and a partner
EXERCISE POSITIONS: Lying, seated, standing, walking
PROGRESSION: Use heavier weights for exercises indicated with asterisk (*). Proceed to Program 5 or 6.

NECK

Resisted Neck #1 .... 8 reps
Resisted Neck #2 .... 8 reps
Resisted Neck #3 .... 8 reps, do both sides

SPINE: UPPER/MID BACK

Side Reverse Fly* .... 8 reps, 2 sets

SPINE: LOWER BACK

Flight .... 8 reps

TORSO STABILIZATION

Partner Push #1 .... 4 reps
Partner Push #2 .... 4 reps
Partner Push #3 .... 4 reps

HIP

Partner Chair Sits .... 8 reps
Lunges* .... 8 reps, 2 sets, each leg
Hip Flexor Stretch .... hold 15 secs, each leg, do twice

WRIST

Wrist Flexion* .... 8 reps, 2 sets, each hand
Wrist Extension* .... 8 reps, 2 sets, each hand

CHEST & ARMS

Press Up .... 8 reps
Full Body Stretch .... hold for 15 secs

ABDOMINALS

In and Up .... 10 reps

BALANCE

Heel Walks .... 10 walks forward, 10 back, 2 sets
One Leg Stand with Knee Bend .... 10 arm swings, each leg
Calf Stretch *with dynaband* .... hold 15 secs, each leg, do twice
Deep Calf Stretch *with dynaband* .... hold 15 secs, each leg, do twice
Ball Catch .... play !

BREATHING

Chest .... do 2 times
Ribcage .... do 2 times
Diaphragm .... do 2 times
Three Dimensional .... do 2 times

PREVENTION · PROGRAM 5

EQUIPMENT NEEDED: Dynaband, dumbbells, chair
EXERCISE POSITIONS: Standing, seated, lying, walking
PROGRESSION: Use heavier resistance. Proceed to Program 6.

SPINE: NECK

Head Lift Back .... 8 reps, 2 sets
Head Lift Side .... 8 reps, do both sides, 2 sets

SPINE: UPPER/MID BACK

Superman .... 8 reps, 2 sets

SPINE: LOWER BACK

Flight .... 8 reps, 2 sets

SPINE: TORSO STABILIZATION

Pelvic Stabilization with Bridge .... 8 reps, 2 sets

HIP

Step Touches *with dynaband* .... 8 step touches, 2 sets
Inner Thigh .... 8 reps, 2 sets, each leg
Jumps .... 10 jumps, 2 sets
Hamstring Stretch .... hold 15 secs, each leg, do twice
Outer Thigh Stretch *with dynaband* .... hold 15 secs, 2 reps, each leg
Inner Thigh Stretch *with dynaband*............ hold 15 secs, 2 reps, each leg

WRIST

Wrist Flexion .... 8 reps, 2 sets, each hand
Wrist Extension .... 8 reps, 2 sets, each hand

CHEST & ARMS

Full Body Hold .... hold 10 secs, 2 sets
Chest Stretch .... hold 15 secs, 2 sets

ABDOMINALS

In and Up .... 10 reps, 2 sets
Reverse Curl .... 10 reps, 2 sets
Side to Side .... 10 times right and left, 2 sets

BALANCE

One Leg Stand with Arm Swing .... swing for 20 seconds

BREATHING

Chest .... do 2 times
Ribcage .... do 2 times
Diaphragm .... do 2 times
Three Dimensional .... do 2 times

PREVENTION · PROGRAM 6

EQUIPMENT NEEDED: Stability ball, stick, ankle weights, dumbbells, chair, and a partner
EXERCISE POSITIONS: Standing, seated, lying, walking, jumping
PROGRESSION: Use heavier resistance for exercises indicated with asterisk (*). Add additional exercises from book.

SPINE: NECK

Resisted Neck #1 .... 8 reps
Resisted Neck #2 .... 8 reps
Resisted Neck #3 .... 8 reps, do both sides

SPINE: UPPER/MID BACK

Goal Post* .... 8 reps, 2 sets

SPINE: LOWER BACK

Trunk Lift *with Stability Ball* .... 8 reps
Arm and Leg Raise *with Stability Ball** ...... 8 reps, switching sides

SPINE: TORSO STABILIZATION

Bridge *with Stability Ball* .... 8 reps
Battle #1 .... once
Battle #2 .... once

HIP

Jumps .... 10 jumps, 3 sets
Squat *with Stability Ball* .... 10 reps, 2 sets
Hip Rotation *on Stability Ball* .... 10 circles, each direction

WRIST

Wrist Flexion* .... 8 reps, 2 sets, each hand
Wrist Extension* .... 8 reps, 2 sets, each hand

CHEST & ARMS

Full Body Hold .... hold for 10 secs, 3 sets
Full Body Stretch .... hold for 15 secs

ABDOMINALS

In and Up .... 10 reps, 2 sets
Reverse Curl *with Stability Ball** .... 10 reps

BALANCE

Ball Catch *on One Leg* .... play!

BREATHING

Chest .... do 2 times
Ribcage .... do 2 times
Diaphragm .... do 2 times
Three Dimensional .... do 2 times

Equipment/Resources

Stability Balls, Tubing, Ankle Weights, Steps

Getfitnow.com
1-800-906-1234
www.getfitnow.com

Fitness Wholesale
1-888-396-7337
www.fwonline.com

Steps

Getfitnow.com
1-800-906-1234
www.getfitnow.com

The Step Company
800-SAYSTEP
www.bodypump.com

Small Balls and Dumbbells

Getfitnow.com
1-800-906-1234
www.getfitnow.com

Sportime
800-444-5700
www.sportime.com

Stability Balls, Dumbbells, Ankle Weights

Getfitnow.com
1-800-906-1234
www.getfitnow.com

Power Systems
800-321-6975
www.power-systems.com

"Boning Up" and Other Publications

Getfitnow.com
1-800-906-1234
www.getfitnow.com

National Osteoporosis Foundation
1232 22nd Street, N.W.
Washington, DC 20037-1292
Tel: 202-223-2226
Fax: 202-223-2237

References

1. Drinkwater, Barbara (1994). Does physical activity play a role in preventing osteoporosis? <u>Research Quarterly for Exercise and Sport, 65</u>(3), 197—206.

2. Gutin, Bernard & Kasper, M. J. (1992). Can vigorous exercise play a role in osteoporosis prevention? A review. <u>Osteoporosis International, 2</u>, 55—59.

3. The American College of Sports Medicine (1995). Position stand on osteoporosis and exercise. <u>Medicine & Science in Sports & Exercise, 27</u>(4), i—vii.

4. Kerr, Deborah, et al (1996). Exercise effects on bone mass in postmenopausal women are site-specific and load-dependent. <u>Journal of Bone and Mineral Research, 11</u>(2), 218—p225.

About the Author

Dianne Daniels has a masters degree in exercise physiology from Columbia University. A former health educator with the New York City Department for the Aging, she has created exercise programs for people from 25–95 years of age. Dianne is on the educational faculty of the American Council on Exercise and New York Sports Clubs, and co-founder of DSY Associates, a partnership which offers lectures and workshops. She has taught academic and practical courses for fitness professionals since 1992, and runs a personal training business in New York City.

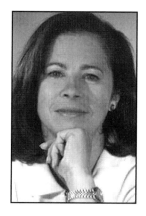